Mutual
Rescue

OCT 0 8

P9-EEG-130

NAPA COUNTY LIBRARY
580 COOMBS STREET
NAPA, CA 94559

Mutual Rescue

How Adopting a Homeless Animal Can Save You, Too

Carol Novello

with Ginny Graves

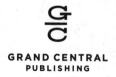

GRAND CENTRAL
PUBLISHING

NEW YORK   BOSTON

Adopting an animal will save a life and enrich yours but adopting the right animal for your lifestyle is key. Reach out to local shelters who can help make a match and assist with safely and appropriately introducing you to a new animal. When approaching an unknown stray animal, practice safety first and call your local shelter for assistance if needed.

Copyright © 2019 by Carol Novello and Humane Society Silicon Valley

All earnings from the sale of this book benefit Mutual Rescue, a national initiative of Humane Society Silicon Valley, a nonprofit corporation.

Cover design by Brian Lemus
Cover photo © Mirko Kuehne / EyeEm
Cover copyright © 2020 by Hachette Book Group, Inc.

Hachette Book Group supports the right to free expression and the value of copyright. The purpose of copyright is to encourage writers and artists to produce the creative works that enrich our culture.

The scanning, uploading, and distribution of this book without permission is a theft of the author's intellectual property. If you would like permission to use material from the book (other than for review purposes), please contact permissions@hbgusa.com. Thank you for your support of the author's rights.

Grand Central Publishing
Hachette Book Group
1290 Avenue of the Americas, New York, NY 10104
grandcentralpublishing.com
twitter.com/grandcentralpub

Originally published in hardcover and ebook in April 2019
First trade paperback edition: April 2020

Grand Central Publishing is a division of Hachette Book Group, Inc. The Grand Central Publishing name and logo is a trademark of Hachette Book Group, Inc.

The publisher is not responsible for websites (or their content) that are not owned by the publisher.

The Hachette Speakers Bureau provides a wide range of authors for speaking events. To find out more, go to www.hachettespeakersbureau.com or call (866) 376-6591.

Library of Congress Cataloging-in-Publication Data
Names: Novello, Carol, author.
Title: Mutual rescue : how adopting a homeless animal can save you, too / by Carol Novello with Ginny Graves.
Description: New York : Grand Central Life & Style, 2019. | Includes bibliographical references.
Identifiers: LCCN 2018044758 | ISBN 9781538713532 (hardcover) | ISBN 9781549175275 (audio download) | ISBN 9781538713556 (ebook)
Subjects: LCSH: Pet adoption—Anecdotes. | Animal shelters—Anecdotes.. | Animal rescue. | Human-animal relationships.
Classification: LCC SF416 .N68 2019 | DDC 636.088/7—dc23
LC record available at https://lccn.loc.gov/2018044758

ISBNs: 978-1-5387-1354-9 (trade paperback), 978-1-5387-1355-6 (ebook)

Printed in the United States of America

LSC-C

10 9 8 7 6 5 4 3 2 1

For all the employees, volunteers, and donors around the world who give their time, energy, heart, and support to the mission of animal welfare:

By saving animals, you're saving humans, too.

For my nieces, Amelia and Julia, who are as beautiful on the inside as they are on the outside.

And for all the animals I've adopted over the years, each of whom, in their own way, has rescued me right back.

Contents

Introduction

From my office at Humane Society Silicon Valley, I look out on a small plot of land dotted with bushes that we call the Community Cat Garden. Inside the fenced space, undomesticated cats, or Carol's Ferals, as my co-workers call them, live until we can find safe homes for them in a barn or garden nursery. These creatures tend to hole up in their condos, like Floridian retirees, emerging predictably at dusk, when their dark profiles are hard to distinguish from the lengthening shadows. My German shepherd rescue, Tess, and I often stare out the window, both hoping to catch a glimpse of one of these reclusive creatures that exist in the netherworld between the average coddled housecat and their large, predatory ancestors who are sometimes sighted in the nearby California hills. The untamed cats' Garbo-esque nature (they "vant to be left alone") is fascinating partly because it stands in stark contrast to most of the pets I've had over the years, who craved my company and care. But they bring to mind another feline from my long-ago past, whose appearance was formative and set the stage for some of the most meaningful decisions I've ever made.

It was the holidays, and my parents and I were shopping at a Christmas tree farm near our home in the Philadelphia suburbs. I was five. The frigid air, alive with the scent of spruce and the tingly anticipation of the season, heightened my sense of purpose: I would find our family the perfect tree. I was eyeing a promising specimen when a slinky shape emerged from beneath its branches. A cat! He walked up to me, and when I knelt down to pet him, his pale amber fur felt like flimsy protection from the cold. He head-butted my knee and began to purr. "Why is he here?" I asked my mom, already smitten. "Do you think he has a home? If he's on his own, can we keep him? *Please???*"

"I'll find out," she said. As I watched her walk away to talk to the farm's owner, my heart was caught in a tug-of-war between hope and disappointment. Based on my five years of experience, the latter appeared far more likely. In our family constellation, my dad and I rotated easily in the same orbit, but my mother always seemed more remote and unreachable. I understood that she loved me in her own way, but it didn't feel the same as it did with my father, whose companionship was like a cozy fire. Warm. Welcoming. Safe. And that's one reason this moment remains firmly rooted in my memory. When my mom returned, she was smiling. "Someone dumped the cat here, so we can keep him," she announced. I was thrilled—and dumbstruck. My mother had said *yes*. More than that, she felt the same tenderness toward this stray that I did. Animals were the crack in her shield that allowed a glimmer of love to break through—a space that enabled her to feel and express love. And, now, miraculously, here she was, after we chose a tree, saying, "Well, come on, Carol, let's get the cat in the car before he freezes to death." For the first time in my young life, I sensed that we might be able to connect. Animals might bridge the divide.

Together, we went to the supermarket and bought our new family member a flounder, which we gift-wrapped and placed under the tree on Christmas morning. All three of us laughed as we watched Nicholas Quattromano (named after St. Nicholas and "four hands" in Italian, a nod to my father's heritage) sniff out his present and shred the paper to uncover—and devour—the fish. Not surprisingly, his rescue ignited my passion for adopting homeless creatures. Rescuing Nick, as we called him, created a way for my mom and me to share the same world. It didn't fix our relationship. But it allowed me to glimpse her softer, more kindhearted side and revealed that we shared something in common.

Even though Nick's initial tentative friendliness turned out to be a calculated gambit to get us to bring him in from the cold—thereafter, he spent the majority of his time atop the refrigerator, safely out of reach of my grasping, cuddling arms—I felt happy that he had a safe home, that he was ours, and that he could depend on us. The seed of my passion for rescuing homeless animals was planted.

Nick was the first of many strays we welcomed into our home over the coming years. His rescue laid the initial stone in my meandering path that led from Harvard Business School to a decade with high-tech software producer Intuit—which set off a search for greater meaning and eventually steered me toward the work I do today as president of our bustling shelter in the heart of Silicon Valley.

Given my lifelong love of animals, accepting the job at Humane Society Silicon Valley was, in my mind, a *fait accompli*. But not everyone saw it that way. Some former colleagues and casual acquaintances, as well as people I met as I began raising money for the organization, didn't understand why someone who had an MBA from Harvard and had run multi-million-dollar businesses for Intuit would veer into animal welfare; others could relate to the impulse to do something philanthropic but didn't get why I wasn't trying to alleviate *human* suffering. Ultimately, they all asked similar versions of the same question: "Why are you helping animals when you could be helping people?"

In response, I'd quote the statistics that spurred my passion for animal welfare: While great strides have been made in saving animals' lives in the United States, more than 6.5 million cats and dogs still enter animal shelters each year—and 1.5 million are euthanized. And of the roughly $410 billion that Americans give to charities, only 3 percent goes to animal-related and environmental causes *combined*. People nodded their heads, and many expressed genuine concern, but I could tell that most weren't fully persuaded. I began to sense that those heartbreaking statistics were only part of the story—that I was missing a deeper truth.

As I groped for a fuller explanation, I started thinking about my mother and how Nick had been the saving grace of our relationship. The tenderness I saw her express toward the creatures that populated our lives showed me she was capable of love, even if she wasn't always able to express it to me in the way I longed for. I still felt saddened by our relationship, but somewhere along the way I realized I could either be resentful and angry for what she didn't give me or grateful for what she did: a devotion to animals that led to my life's purpose. I chose the latter. As I thought more about what animals have meant in my life—how they've given me hope when I was despondent, laughter when I was stressed, companionship when I was lonely—as well as the lives of nearly every pet owner I know, I finally saw it—the hidden "why" of animal rescue: By helping animals I *am* helping people—helping them heal their own pain, find greater purpose, and discover more sources of joy.

The human race is definitely in need of help. The magnitude of misery, even in our prosperous country, is mind-boggling. Sixteen million adults in the United States struggle with depression. About 8 million adults in any given year have post-traumatic stress disorder. Twenty-nine million are diagnosed with diabetes, and an estimated 8 million have it but don't yet know it. Meanwhile, nearly 40 percent of people are obese. And that's not counting the grieving, heartbroken, sedentary masses who may not be diagnosable but are struggling and hurting nonetheless. But there's hope for a healthier future, and what leads us toward it may very well have four legs and a tail. Companion animals can help relieve a range of troubles— and as I and my writing collaborator, Ginny Graves, explain in the chapters ahead, there's scientific research that proves it. The data affirming animals' positive effects on human health is so persuasive that 60 percent of doctors in a recent survey said they prescribe pet adoption, and a staggering 97 percent believe pet ownership provides health benefits. While this research is applicable to animals in general—regardless of whether they were rescued or not—giving a shelter animal a home confers a special kind of restorative grace.

Naturally, I'm biased toward encouraging people to adopt shelter pets. But I believe that showing benevolence for a homeless creature fertilizes the seeds of kindness, generosity, and compassion that exist inside us, spurring those qualities to put down roots and thrive. It grounds us in love.

People facing serious challenges often benefit profoundly from adopting an animal, but pets can enrich *anyone's* busy life. They also come with their share of demands and headaches, of course, as anyone who has stepped in warm dog barf at four a.m. can testify. But caring for another creature, and having someone who depends on you, can be its own kind of blessing, adding dimension and meaning to the daily routine. And beyond the hassles, most people who adopt an animal find so much reward.

Cats and dogs inject contentment, warmth, and goofy little hits of delight into our days that distract us from our worries, keep us grounded in the here and now, and remind us what matters— including the fact that a grubby tennis ball or ratty ball of yarn can be a source of real joy. My cat, Wilbur, a master prankster whom I adopted when I was thirty, revealed the wonder of kitchen drawers. He would pull out a bottom drawer, crawl behind it, claw his way up the rear of the cabinet, and emerge out the top drawer, like Houdini popping to the surface after being shackled in an underwater crate. Wilbur would look at me like, *"Ta-da! Pretty cool, huh?"* It never failed to make me laugh—and ease the stress of work. Wilbur was an antidepressant and anxiety cure in a single furry package.

In studies with a variety of types of people, the same story emerges. Interacting with an animal can lift mood, increase well-being, and facilitate the ability to communicate and connect. Given the rampant ill health, emotional and physical, in our culture, that's actually a profoundly hopeful, and radically important, finding. After accepting my role at Humane Society Silicon Valley, I began finding evidence of the life-changing impact of pets everywhere, and the more stories I heard about people who'd regained their vitality and flourished after adopting a cat or dog, the more urgently

I felt the need to share them. People needed to know that rescuing an animal doesn't mean ignoring humanity's woes; it's a vital part of the solution!

In 2015, a board member introduced me to David Whitman, a storyteller and creative producer, who helped me come up with a way to spread the word about the transformative power of adopting an animal. He coined the phrase "mutual rescue" and suggested we make short films of people whose lives have been dramatically bettered by rescuing an animal. As it happened, I had the perfect candidate already in mind. About a year before, we had received a letter from an obese man who told us he'd become vastly healthier after adopting an overweight dog from our shelter. We made his journey the subject of our first film, hoping it would reach enough people to inspire others across the country to submit their own stories for consideration and encourage people to adopt shelter animals. We had no idea what we were in for. *Eric & Peety*, that first short film, caught fire and has now been viewed more than 100 million times in more than forty countries.

We were *flooded* with story submissions from people who'd been depressed, suicidal, diabetic, broken, homeless, lonely, and more—all of whom had moving, uplifting stories about how their rescue pets had saved them. We turned four of their redemptive stories into short films—and watched this international phenomenon flourish. *Kylie & Liza*, our second film, released in early 2017, tells the story of an effervescent twelve-year-old girl battling lethal bone cancer and the kitten she adopts, who, after her death, became a vital source of solace for her grieving mom. We released three more films later that year, and collectively those four films have garnered more than 35 million views to date.

The films struck a chord because they depict the essence of mutual rescue. But as we dug deeper into our trove of anecdotes, I realized the full story of what happens when a human adopts an animal can't be told in a five-minute film. One of the truly astonishing aspects of this phenomenon is that the uplifting effect often spreads *beyond* the person who adopts a stray. Take my experience with Wilbur and his feline brother, Wiley, who was a total love bug with his own sweet charisma. By buoying me up and bolstering my resilience, those two helped me be a more genial and compassionate leader at work, which created a collaborative environment that allowed my team to feel more empowered and function more effectively. In other words, two goofball cats helped set off a mini upward spiral of positive energy. And that's just one small example of something that happens routinely when a person rescues an animal: The meaningful bond humans often form with their pets can foster a deep sense of well-being that allows them to embrace life and love more fully, and they may inspire others to do the same.

A Harvard study tracking the lives of 238 men since 1938 has found that close relationships, more than money or success, are what make us happy. George Vaillant, who led the study from 1972 to 2004, wrote that there are two pillars of this deep and enduring happiness: "One is love," he says. "The other is finding a way of coping with life that does not push love away." Rescue animals are a coping mechanism that *draws love in*—increasing the odds that we can *radiate love out*. And when one person becomes more upbeat, the feeling can spread to others, according to a separate group of Harvard researchers. Their fascinating studies revealed that having a happy friend who lives within a mile increases the probability that you will be happy, too—and that bliss often spreads to neighbors, nearby siblings, and spouses. In other words, the joy one person generates from adopting an animal can be contagious.

I've come to think of this phenomenon as the "rescue effect," because adopting an animal can create ripples of well-being that impact concentric circles of people—sometimes even total strangers. The idea was inspired by "the butterfly effect," a scientific phenomenon that shows, in essence, that the flap of a butterfly's wings in Australia can set enough molecules of air in motion to create a tornado in Kansas. Put simply: Small changes can have surprisingly large consequences.

In the following chapters, we reveal the countless ways this plays out in real people's lives. We start with the Heart section, where you'll meet people whose rescue animals have helped them face inconceivable trauma and grief and provided the strength, courage, and wisdom they needed to find their way forward. In the Body section, we share stories of people who've learned that adopting a cat or dog can not only help them become healthier but also help them cope with and recover from physical illnesses and injuries and show them how to thrive in spite of their disabilities—and experience more joy. In Mind, you'll see how rescue animals can actually save people coping with anxiety, depression, and post-traumatic stress disorder (PTSD), offering them hope, helping them create healthier patterns of thought, and leading them toward lives filled with meaning and compassion. But nearly every story has all three elements—heart, mind, *and* body—a graphic demonstration of the expansive and multifaceted impact of rescuing an animal. And people in these narratives aren't the only ones who benefit; the animals do, too, in ways that are surprising, tender, and sometimes profound.

Finally, in Connection, we reveal how pets can strengthen our relationships with the people we love, how we can bond deeply with many types of animals, not just cats and dogs, and how, when rescue pets make people healthier and happier, something remarkable can happen: Their hearts mended, these humans often go on to make positive contributions to the world and pay forward the love and healing they received. Some find a deeper sense of purpose, others develop a stronger understanding of who they are and why they're here, and some even discover a renewed sense of their own personal faith or relationship with something divine, however they define it.

The stories and research in this book reveal what I know to be true: Rescue pets can help us evolve as people, because they give us a safe way to practice opening our hearts, and once we learn how to be more open and empathetic with pets, we can become more compassionate with ourselves, better at being tender with others—and more inspired to contribute to humanity.

Animals can bring us face-to-face with both our flaws and our deeper potential. They can train us to be more reliable and responsible. They can help us overcome our shortcomings and set us on the road to becoming our *best* selves—loving, nurturing, caring, giving. And by presenting us with the opportunity to learn and grow, they offer us the chance to become a source of light and hope for humankind. As we teach them to heel, they show us how to *heal*.

SECTION I

HEART

I

Finding Courage

Pets as Secure Bases and Safe Havens

On the morning of February 28, 2018, Grace Briden's mom drove her and her sister to high school, as usual. But that was the only thing ordinary about the day. Grace was a sophomore at Marjory Stoneman Douglas High School in Parkland, Florida, and two weeks before, one teacher, two coaches, and fourteen of her classmates, including one of Grace's friends, had been shot and killed at the school. During the ordeal, Grace had hidden in a classroom with thirty other students for three and a half hours, crying and praying, not knowing where the gunman was, if her sister was safe, or if any of them would make it out of the school alive. Ever since, she'd been plagued by flashbacks and nightmares of hunkering down in that room, of her friends sobbing, and of the paralyzing fear she felt while waiting to see if they were going to live or die. "I never wanted to set foot in that school again. I was sure I'd have a panic attack if I went on campus. I didn't know if I could get through it," she says.

Even so, there she was, making her way through the throng of media, heavily armed police officers, well-wishers, and parents on the first day Stoneman Douglas reopened. The fence was adorned with flowers, cards, candles, and memorials. The crowd cheered as the students walked in. "I know they were trying to be supportive, but I didn't like the fanfare," she says. "I was super anxious, because I thought there might be another shooting."

While Grace was outside braving the crowd, inside the school, Marni Bellavia, a dog trainer and manager of the Animal Assisted Therapy program at Humane Society of Broward County, was awaiting the students' arrival near the roped-off building where the shooting occurred. She'd brought her mini-Australian shepherd rescue, Karma, a trained therapy dog, as well as her team of twenty volunteers and their therapy dogs, all rescues, to comfort the students. Six years before, Karma, just a one-year-old puppy, had been found wandering the streets in a small town in Mississippi. She was dangerously overweight but sweet and friendly. When her rescuers called the number on her tag, her owners said they didn't want her back. The local shelter sent Karma to Humane Society of Broward County—facilities often handle overpopulation by transferring animals to locations with higher demand—where Marni adopted her. By the time Karma was two, she was certified as a therapy animal. She'd worked with the elderly, kids with autism, and people with traumatic brain injuries, but, prior to the Stoneman Douglas shooting, she'd never comforted trauma victims. "I knew she'd do great," Marni says. "She's extraordinarily attentive to people, loves to give and receive affection, and has an innate sense of who needs her the most."

As Grace approached the building where the shooting occurred, tears began welling in her eyes, and she wanted nothing more than to turn around and go home. "My friends were saying don't look over there," she says. "Then out of the corner of my eye, I saw Karma. She was so adorable I ran up to her and started petting her. She snuggled into me, and something changed inside me. Ever since the shooting, I'd been depressed. My heart felt so heavy. But Karma lifted my heart. She broke through the sadness and gave me something good to focus on. And she didn't just say hi and walk away, like dogs sometimes do. She stayed with me. She licked my hand.

She let me pet her. She gave me the chance to calm down. I don't know if she knew how much comfort I felt. But she gave me the courage to get through the day."

From then on, Grace sought out Karma and the other therapy dogs every chance she got. "I talked to therapists, but the dogs were the only reason I was able to go to school. The shooting changed me. I didn't think I'd ever smile or be happy again. But the dogs' attention and love made me see there was still good in the world. They were the key to helping me come back to my new self," she says.

Like Grace, sixteen-year-old Jonathan Sullivan dreaded going back to Stoneman Douglas. He had been in his fourth period ceramics class when the fire alarm went off on February fourteenth, the day of the shooting. As his class filed outside, word began to spread that there was a shooter in the freshman building. "I saw a Snapchat video of a kid huddled on the floor of a classroom, with the sound of gunshots in the background, and I just started running," says Jonathan.

He scrambled over a nearby chain-link fence, then ran toward the apartment where he and his dad, Joe, lived, about a quarter mile from the school. The streets were already jammed with empty cars, abandoned by desperate parents trying to get to their kids, and hundreds of uniformed officers carrying guns. "It felt like a war zone," says Jonathan. When he reached the roundabout near their home, his dad, frantic with worry, was there waiting. "I just kept thinking, 'Let Johnny be okay,'" recalls Joe. "Seeing him was the happiest moment of my life. We hugged each other, and I said, 'Let's go home.'"

But the young man who had left home that morning wasn't the same one who shuffled into their apartment that afternoon. "Every time I closed my eyes to go to sleep, the day of the shooting would start running through my mind," says Jonathan. "I'd put myself in the shoes of the kids who got shot. I couldn't get those thoughts out of my head, so I wasn't able to sleep." Jonathan was withdrawn, too. Even Joe couldn't reach him. "I've been a single dad since Johnny was three, and we've always been really close," says Joe. "But he was just sort of lost. I couldn't blame him. I'm an adult, and I didn't know how to cope with this kind of tragedy."

When Jonathan got home from that first day back at school, however, Joe noticed a change. "All he talked about was the comfort dogs," Joe says. "After the second day, he came home and said, 'I think I need a dog.'"

That night, Joe called 100+ Abandoned Dogs of Everglades Florida Rescue and learned there was a litter of puppies at a foster home not far from his apartment. Several weeks before, a police officer had found the flea-infested puppies in the backyard of a home in Miami. The puppies' parents were chained in the yard, and their stomachs were swollen nearly to the point of bursting, after being fed a diet of raw beans and rice. The officer took the litter to the rescue group, who nursed them back to health.

"Johnny and I went to see them, and one puppy just rolled over and wanted belly rubs. We fell in love with him," says Joe. "The rescue organization waived the fees and gave us dog food. I will always be grateful for their generosity and how sensitive they were to Johnny's situation."

Jonathan named his new puppy Ajax. "He was friendly and loving and so excited to see me every day. Just knowing that he'd be waiting for me when I came home from school made me feel better," he says. "Friends and classmates came over every day so they could hang out with Ajax, too. When we were sitting around playing with the dog, kids would start opening up about what happened. Ajax softened the atmosphere and made us all feel okay about talking about stuff. He helped lots of kids feel better."

Joe was astonished by the effect the puppy had on his son. "Johnny went from not sleeping and not wanting to talk about anything to communicating again and feeling more like his old self," he says. "This was a puppy, not some trained service dog, but he always seemed to know just what we needed. I don't know how we would have made it through that time without Ajax."

The puppy, Jonathan says, made them feel safe. "Not that Ajax is a guard dog. Far from it. But with him by my side, I was able to sleep. And knowing that he was relying on me helped me feel stronger," Jonathan says, adding, "I used to hear about school shootings and wonder what that would be like. Now I know. It's even worse than you think. It messes you up. But Ajax and I developed this bond. Being with him made me feel like I could handle life again."

Cats and Dogs Can Enlarge Our Capacity for Courage

By the time of the Parkland shooting, I'd been collecting stories of people who'd been saved by rescue pets for several years. I'd heard hundreds of stories that inspired me and moved me to tears, and I was overwhelmed by the diverse and often miraculous ways rescuing an animal can save a person, too. But hearing about Grace and Jonathan left me short of breath.

I've faced heartbreak and lost loved ones I miss to this day. But I couldn't imagine what it would feel like to endure such a needless tragedy, nor could I conceive of the courage it must have taken the students—much less the families in Parkland who lost daughters and sons and loved ones—to move forward in its aftermath. It made me think of the definition of courage from Brené Brown, author and research professor at the University of Houston's Graduate College of Social Work: "Courage is a heart word. The root of the word courage is cor—the Latin word for heart. In one of its earliest forms, the word courage meant 'To speak one's mind by telling all one's heart.' Over time, this definition has changed, and today, we typically associate courage with heroic and brave deeds. But in my opinion, this definition fails to recognize the inner strength and level of commitment required for us to actually speak honestly and openly about who we are and about our experience good and bad. Speaking from our hearts is what I think of as 'ordinary courage.'"

In the aftermath of the shooting, Grace and Jonathan needed both bravery and ordinary courage—bravery to show up for school every day and ordinary courage to open up and cope with what had happened. And the humans involved weren't the only ones whose circumstances required mettle. Imagine the stoutness of heart Karma and Ajax, neglected and abandoned, would've had to call upon to survive. When their rescuers delivered them to the safety of their respective shelters, they actually saved numerous lives. Meeting Karma was pivotal for Grace's healing—and untold numbers of others as well. And adopting Ajax was the choice that shored up Jonathan's nerve and allowed both him and Joe to face the horror of what had happened and brave whatever came next.

And it's not just dogs that can give traumatized people strength. Nichole Stone, twenty-five, of Salem, Oregon, was at the Las Vegas Route 91 Harvest music festival in September 2017, when a gunman opened fire on the crowd. "I'm not sure what would have happened to me afterward if it hadn't been for my cat, Connor," she says. When she'd adopted him as a kitten in June 2014 from Best Friends Animal Society in Mission Hills, California, he was scrawny and tiny, with a crooked tail and disheveled fur. "He licked my face and I knew he was the one," she says. After the shooting, Connor seemed to sense that Nichole needed extra attention. "I'd wake up from a dream about the shooting that was so real it felt like I was there all over again. Connor would lick my face and remind me I was home and safe. I have a lot of guilt since the concert. Why am I still here when fifty-eight people didn't come home that weekend? But I can't let that break me, because I can't leave my little beast. He's given me the strength to get through it."

The circumstances of Grace's, Jonathan's, and Nichole's experiences were extraordinary. But we all come up against challenges that require us to take a stand or speak up or summon a firm sense of resolve, and the support we get from loved ones can steel us to face down trials large and small. If our human network frays or falls short, however—or we fail to reach out for help—we can become isolated. Alone, our worry-prone minds, which evolved over millennia to scan for threats, can fall prey to anxiety, depression, anger, fear, and insecurity. At those dark and withdrawn times, our kinship with pets can be the bedrock that anchors us and helps us move fearlessly forward.

How Bonding With Our Pets Helps Us Be Brave

In my years at Humane Society Silicon Valley, I've been fortunate to witness remarkable examples of human-animal synergy a number of times, but after hearing Nichole's and the Stoneman Douglas students' stories I needed to know: *How* does that type of mutual rescue happen? Why did interacting with animals help Grace, Jonathan, and Nichole feel brave? What do pets do for us that amplifies our capacity for courage?

The simplest answer is the one we all think of first: unconditional love. Whether the creature curled up at your feet is a regal Persian you fell for at your local shelter or a wounded pit bull found wandering the streets, you already know that rescue animals can serve as an unwavering source of affection—and being loved is a source of power. But love is only part of the story. As you'll read below, research shows that something deeper and less well recognized happens when we bring a pet into our home, and it stems not just from what we get from our animals but from what we become capable of *giving* when we experience the safety and security their love provides. Our rescue pets' affection can mobilize our strength; our love for them helps us turn our minds from fear to fortitude, so we're staunch enough to be a source of strength, not only for ourselves but for others, too.

At Austria's esteemed Wolf Science Center, Kurt Kotrschal, a biologist, and his colleagues (which include nearly twenty timber wolves and fifteen mutts rescued from Hungarian animal shelters) have spent the past decade delving into the thriving research area of human-animal attachment, trying to tease apart the behavioral nuances and biological underpinnings of our mysterious ability to love creatures of different species. When we caught up with

Kotrschal, who is also a professor in the department of behavioral biology at the University of Vienna, he explained over the phone that in order to grasp the full impact of our relationships with pets, we first need to understand how we bond with people—and the place to start is with attachment theory, a psychological concept developed in the 1970s to describe the most fundamental of our evolutionary relationships: the infant-parent bond. "This bond developed very early in our evolution to keep mothers and their offspring physically close and protect babies from predators," Kotrschal told us. "As a result, the young of many species are wired to want to be near their mothers and to look at them as a reliable source of safety and comfort."

Attachment doesn't just keep infants physically safe. It provides emotional security as well. Dozens of studies of human infants and children have shown that those who form secure attachments to their parents—who have learned to trust that their guardians will care for them and protect them from harm—are better able to develop the confidence they need to explore their environments, cultivate friendships, venture ever farther afield, and, eventually, flourish as independent adults.

Healthy attachments allow children to see the world as a positive place and become resilient enough to rebound from adversity. They help children develop, among other things, courage. And those reliable bonds aren't just important for the young. We need them, and continue to forge them, throughout our lives with friends and romantic partners—relationships we trust and rely on for emotional support and comfort. Moreover, Kotrschal says, the bond we form with our pets is remarkably similar.

There's a reason so many of us find it completely natural to think of our pets as family members. The basis for the mother-infant bond and all the important attachments that follow in its wake—including with animals—is largely biological. Bonding, attachment, caregiving, and social relationships are driven, on the most basic level, by ancient structures in the brain. This "social network," as biologists call it, may have developed four hundred fifty million years ago in an ancestor that all mammals share. "This handful of brain regions hasn't changed much in structure and function over the past five hundred million years, and it's the basis for instinctive social behavior in humans and cats and dogs, as well as many other species," says Kotrschal. From the moment you adopt an animal, you begin to mobilize this ancient cognitive machinery designed to protect our species by stimulating attachment.

Not everyone successfully bonds with their pets. We all know people for whom adoptions haven't worked out, or who become attached in an unhealthy way, allowing a dog or cat to serve as a stand-in for vital human connections in their lives. But having seen thousands of rescue animals find happy homes, I know that the majority of people form deep ties with their new companions—and those relationships often become a mainstay of joy, camaraderie, safety, and courage.

Surprising Things Happen When You Become Attached to a Pet

Several years ago, leading researchers in the attachment research field from the University of California at Davis and Israel's Inter-disciplinary Center collaborated on two groundbreaking studies that illuminate how deeply we bond with our pets—and reveal the potentially meaningful role those bonds can play in our lives. In the first, the researchers assessed 165 pet owners' attachment to their cats or dogs with a questionnaire designed to determine if they had a healthy bond. Then they divided the participants into three groups and asked them to list all their current personal life goals—their hopes and dreams for the future—and rate the likelihood of achieving each goal on a seven-point scale. One group had their pet in the room with them while they completed the task; the second group was prompted through a writing exercise to think about their absent pets while they wrote about their goals; and a third group worked on the assignment alone, after being cued with a writing exercise to think about a person they knew but weren't close to.

The results: Among participants who were securely attached to their pets, being with their animals—or even just thinking about them—allowed them to list more personal goals and express more confidence in their ability to meet them. Participants were able to engage in a richer exploration of their goals because their pets served as a "secure base," just as human attachment figures can—a type of support that helps you feel more comfortable and confident about trying new things, pursuing goals, engaging in challenging activities, and taking reasonable risks.

The same researchers conducted a second trial designed to assess whether a dog or cat can serve as a "safe haven," another indispensable type of support that gives us a sense of comfort, reassurance, and protection in times of danger or distress, just as a good friend or close family member would. Having an ally (human or animal) who provides a safe haven helps you cope more effectively with stressful life events and can actually lead to better physical and mental health. In this study, the researchers enlisted a new set of 120 participants and divided them into the same three groups as before (one had their pets with them, the second just thought about their pets, and the third didn't have a pet present and thought about a random person). Then each group completed a particularly tricky timed word test specifically designed to elicit feelings of failure and frustration. Researchers took participants' blood pressure before the challenge as well as during the test.

When they crunched the numbers, the results were remarkable. Compared to people in the no-pet condition, those whose pets were in the room with them, or who merely thought about their cat or dog, were more likely to say the test felt like a challenge rather than a threat, and also remained calmer, with diastolic and systolic blood pressure that was several points lower.

Together, the studies indicate that pets, like supportive friends and loved ones, provide their owners with a secure base from which they can explore the world, pursue ambitions, and grow as people, and also serve as a safe haven that can provide comfort and soothe their distress in times of need. Think about that: Our pets can help us stay calmer in the face of stress and more confident about our ability to attain life goals. The same furry characters who track mud on the carpet, shred armchairs, chew shoes, and leave filaments of fur on practically everything we own also provide a vital sense of emotional security that is the wellspring for our ability to function bravely in the world.

Reams of research show that healthy attachments are vital to our well-being. And attachment is just the first phase in the natural arc of every single important relationship in our lives—an arc that follows a path from attachment and bonding to separation, loss, and the painful process of bereavement. From there, if we move through the sadness and don't start closing ourselves off, we're able to form new attachments and repeat the process all over, from happiness to heartbreak and back again. By virtue of animals' ability to show us unfiltered affection and loyalty—and their heartbreakingly short life spans—they give us a safe way to practice and hone our ability to move through the ups and downs of the bonding cycle. As a result, our uncomplicated relationships with cats and dogs help us become better at meeting people, loving deeply, coping with loss and grief and, afterward, establishing new relationships that allow us to reclaim joy and fearlessly entrust our hearts to another. They help us more courageously embrace *life*.

A Fearful Dog Offers a Lesson in Bravery

Over the years, I've seen this bolstering effect of pets play out in many different ways. Two years before I heard Grace's and Jonathan's stories, another moving anecdote arrived in my inbox—this one featuring Nigel, a timid ninety-pound black Lab mix, who gave Amanda Ellis Bronowski, twenty-nine, of Moscow, Idaho, the conviction to confront a nightmare that was unfolding under her own roof.

At nineteen, Amanda began dating a handsome, charming man, and the first six months of their relationship were fairy-tale perfect. "He was attentive and sweet. He'd cook me dinner and surprise me with little gifts," she says. Then, disturbing cracks began to appear. When she made plans with her friends, he'd question where she was going and whom she was going to be with. Soon, the questions escalated to accusations of flirting, of cheating. He picked fights and called her names. *Slut. Whore. Crazy bitch.* "Every time he got out of control, he'd end up crying and apologizing, and he always had a different excuse: He's depressed, he's suicidal, he has trust issues because his old girlfriend cheated on him," she says. "He knew the right story to get me to stay."

Amanda never so much as hinted at his bad behavior to anyone. She was too ashamed—and kept hoping he'd change. Besides, by the time they'd been together three years, she had almost no close friends left. "He got so stressed every time I went out; it was easier to just do things with him," she says. The one true ally who was with her through it all: Nigel. Amanda's mom had found the big black stray when she was hiking not far from her home in the summer of 2007. They couldn't find anyone who had lost a dog. After reading that dogs and cats with black fur linger the longest in shelters—their dark features are less distinct than lighter-colored animals', which can make it seem harder at first to create an emotional connection—she decided to keep him, a decision that delighted Amanda, who was home from her freshman year of college at the time.

"I bonded with Nigel from moment one. He followed me everywhere," she says. The big, kindhearted stray turned out to be afraid of *everything*—garbage cans, bicycles, vacuums, thunder. "He stole my heart because he was just this sweet, cowardly dog," says Amanda. When she moved in with her boyfriend a year later, Nigel came, too. "He saw it all—the arguments, the belittling, the making up. During that time, Nigel became my best friend. He was always there when I needed comfort," she says.

One night Amanda and her boyfriend began arguing over

something trivial—Amanda doesn't even remember what triggered the spat—and she told him she was leaving. "I was lying on our bed with Nigel. My boyfriend was standing in the doorway—and he went ballistic. He began yelling, then grabbed the nightstand and threw it across the room," recalls Amanda. "When he turned around, Nigel was standing over my body, staring intently at him. He was shaking like a leaf and his tail was tucked between his legs, but he didn't break eye contact, and his body language was clear. He was saying, 'If you touch her, you'll regret it.' Even though he was terrified, he was prepared to defend me."

In that moment, Amanda finally saw her situation clearly. "I saw my boyfriend from Nigel's perspective, and I was forced to admit something I'd been in denial about for years: I was in an abusive relationship," she says. "I suddenly couldn't believe I'd put either Nigel or myself in such danger. I grabbed his leash and a laundry basket full of clean clothes, and he and I walked out the door. But the truth is, I might have gone back, because my self-esteem was so low. When a loved one abuses you, it makes you feel like you're not a valuable, worthy human being. But I kept thinking of that moment when Nigel stood over me, and that image helped me stay strong. He helped me find the courage to stay away and rebuild my life and my self-confidence."

It's like Brené Brown says: "Courage is contagious. Every time we choose courage, we make everyone around us a little better and the world a little braver."

If ever a situation calls for bravery, it's leaving an abusive relationship. One in four women in the United States are victims of physical violence at the hands of their partners, and nearly twice as many endure psychological abuse—and the risk of violence skyrockets when women threaten to leave. All types of abuse can erode victims' self-esteem and lead to depression, but researchers at California State University found that emotional violence may cause even deeper wounds than physical abuse. Emotional cruelty slowly chips away at the very core of who you are. At a certain point, some victims no longer trust themselves to be able to function outside the unhealthy relationship, one reason they don't leave. But with an animal by their side, victims are often better able to maintain their self-esteem and emotional stability, and sometimes have a potent stimulus to leave.

Curious to learn more about how this might work, we contacted Amy Fitzgerald, a researcher at the University of Windsor in Canada who has undertaken a number of studies on the role animals play in the lives of domestic violence victims. She told us she began thinking about the topic when she was volunteering at an animal shelter, where she processed the paperwork for people relinquishing animals. "Quite a few women said they had to get rid of their pets because their partners were threatening or harming the animals, so for my master's thesis I decided to study it," she says.

After conducting in-depth interviews with twenty-six domestic abuse survivors, Fitzgerald found that, just as Nigel did for Amanda, pets frequently protect women from their abusers by meowing, barking, or even attacking the abuser. Animals also shield women emotionally, Fitzgerald told us—even, in some cases, preventing victims from taking their own lives. "Their pets were often their lifeline—the companionship and emotional support that pulled them through."

Dogs and cats may be especially well suited to support abused women for a number of reasons. "They don't judge, and they're uniquely able to offer comfort, often when no one else could, or would," she explains. "For some women, their pets became an integral part of their ability to survive and sometimes were the motivation for leaving the relationship."

At the same time, animals can also be the reason some women stay. Research shows that about a third of domestic violence victims don't leave because they can't find a women's shelter to go to that accepts pets. They're afraid of what will happen to their cats or dogs if they leave them behind, since abusers often see pets as a way to threaten, manipulate, and, by harming the animals, heap more abuse on their victims. But animal shelters are becoming more aware of the problem and trying to help. Our Ani-Safe program at Humane Society Silicon Valley offers accommodations for the pets of domestic violence victims—and the Animal Welfare Institute has a searchable database of rescue facilities across the country that have similar options. (Go to awionline.org/safe-havens. Also, additional resources can be found at safeplaceforpets.org and redrover.org.) Still, more work needs to be done to address the problem. "Pets are an overlooked, but incredibly important, piece of the domestic violence equation," says Fitzgerald. "Battered women shelters and support groups are aware of the problem, which is good, but most don't ask about pets in any formal way. We hope that by raising awareness we can solve that problem."

Rescue Pets and the Biology of Bonding

Animals can also bolster us through less dramatic circumstances by providing what I think of as "small c" courage. It's not the type of superhuman valor you need in life-or-death circumstances. It's the chutzpah we call upon routinely to meet everyday challenges. In the introduction, I told the story of my cat, Wilbur, and his fondness for kitchen drawers. But Wilbur's antics were more than just amusing. His presence along with Wiley's, my other cat, were essential to my well-being. I was living in Santa Rosa, California, and running a newly acquired company for Intuit—a two-hour drive from friends and a five-hour flight from family. I'd underestimated just how hard that would be. I was lonely, stressed, and working long hours, with little time to meet new people. But I'd made a professional commitment to turn this company around and had to find some way to cope.

One lonely night, I was sitting on the sofa. Wilbur was nestled in the crook of my arm and Wiley was purring on my lap when it occurred to me: I was staying afloat in large part because of them. Yes, I was stressed and lonely. But I woke up every morning and came home every night to two loyal felines, who knew nothing, and cared even less, about balance sheets. Their expertise lay in a very human, and vital, contact sport: snuggling. As important, they made me laugh, offered companionship, and gave me the chance to nurture living creatures instead of bottom lines. By doing so, they kept me centered and kept me sane.

Because my affection for Wilbur and Wiley was a form of healthy attachment, being with them, petting them, nuzzling them, and singing made-up songs to them didn't just lift me emotionally; it affected me physically, says Kotrschal. Deep under my skin, a chemical that's associated with bonding and love was surging through my body. We'll talk more about this in coming chapters, but being with pets is profoundly grounding partly because it triggers the release of oxytocin, the same hormone that's released when moms breast-feed their newborns and the most important hormone involved in the brain's primitive social network. Oxytocin is the glue that cements that first, pivotal relationship—and it's at work, too, when we're falling in love. It's found in most mammals, not just humans. And because it encourages bonding, it pushes us to ally ourselves with "safe" others, which gives us the courage to function in uncertain and trying circumstances.

The sense of safety Grace and the other traumatized students at Stoneman Douglas felt as they snuggled and bonded with Karma was likely the result of oxytocin. And when Ajax rolled over for a belly rub and gazed into Jonathan's eyes, a burst of oxytocin almost certainly surged through his system (and probably Ajax's) as well; as their relationship deepened, so, too, did oxytocin's effects, making Jonathan feel secure and restoring his faith in himself.

Like so many others who have adopted rescue animals during difficult moments, these traumatized young people learned something surprising: The secure relationship we develop with our pets can be the foundation that makes it possible for us to process our pain rather than be consumed by it, and sometimes even be courageous enough to give the gift of strength to others.

Nigel showed Amanda how to summon the nerve to say "No more" and gave her the confidence to give love another chance. She reconnected with a man she had known through work. He was kind, supportive, patient, calm. When he proposed, she happily said yes. "He adores me and loves and appreciates the dog that changed my life as much as I do," she says. Ajax helped Jonathan regain his equilibrium, reconnect with friends and family, and join his fellow Parkland students in speaking out about gun violence. Grace made key chains and sold them to raise funds both for the victims of the Marjory Stoneman Douglas shooting and for the animal-assisted therapy program at Humane Society of Broward County. And Karma's remarkable ability to comfort the traumatized Stoneman Douglas students inspired Marni Bellavia, the manager of that animal-assisted therapy program, to start a state-of-the-art initiative at the shelter. Known as Canines for Community Resilience, the therapy teams are undergoing training with the police and fire departments and local hospitals to help them act as first responders in a range of traumatic situations.

Brené Brown is right: Courage *is* contagious. And rescue animals, survivors one and all, can pass it on to us. We just need to be bold enough to embrace it.

2

Building Trust

Animals and the Biochemistry of Bonding

Kat Noe was sitting at an outdoor table with a dozen people at a packed bar in Athens, Georgia, her hometown, when a big, black dog made her way across the patio, walked straight over to Kat's chair, and placed her head in her lap. While Kat petted the dog, the man holding the other end of the long, retractable leash walked up. It was Jim, another local, who explained that he'd seen the friendly pup wandering the streets but wasn't in a position to give her a home. "So, do you want her?" he asked. Kat's knee-jerk response: *No way.* "I was twenty-four and just barely surviving," she says. "I made a thousand dollars a month working in a grocery store deli, I was living in a tiny, windowless room in a house with one other person and partying into the wee hours every night."

Kat's troubles began when she was a teenager. "I'd been an honor student and close to my parents in middle school. But then I started partying and hanging with a rough crowd and was in and out of a juvenile detention center. When my parents discovered I was gay, I felt unwelcome at home," she recalls. "There was so much tension that when I was fifteen I hopped a freight train and disappeared." Shortly thereafter, she received devastating news: The girlfriend she'd left behind had hanged herself. "I knew it wasn't my fault, but as a teenager you still blame yourself."

With no support system nearby, she was left to grapple with the loss on her own. She felt too estranged from her parents to go home. So for four years she wandered the country—a young girl, homeless and alone. "I drank and did drugs. I got piercings and tattoos. I was mugged and sexually assaulted. I had some good times, too, but I learned not to trust anyone. I believed that everyone was going to judge me or leave me or die."

By the time she was in her twenties, Kat says, it felt easier to live off the grid and let herself spiral downward than allow someone into her world and risk getting hurt. But as she sat in the bar that night with an unfamiliar dog's head in her lap, the brazen sweetness of the gentle canine's gesture stirred something in Kat she thought she'd long ago stamped out. "I looked into her sparkly brown eyes, and it was like this dog was saying, 'Stop it. You're better than all this.' I knew she had something to teach me, and I knew I had to listen."

Jim told Kat that the young dog was all but homeless herself—abandoned by her original owner, a college student, and now in the care of her elderly great-grandmother, who let the neglected canine roam. Jim had offered to try and find the dog a new home. "She was alone like me, but she wasn't a loner. She didn't choose her solitary life, and she seemed to crave connection," says Kat. "When I tried to shoo her away, she rolled her eyes at me, like, 'Yeah, right. That's not going to happen.'" By the end of the evening, Jim convinced Kat to meet him and the dog in the park the next day. The meeting lasted less than five minutes. "The dog looked up at me with these hopeful eyes, and I thought about how, of all the people in the bar, she had put her head in my lap. I knew I had to take her," says Kat.

Even so, their first months together weren't easy. "I was so wary of getting close to anyone that I couldn't even name her for several weeks. Then one day I was shopping for wine and realized she was sassy and sharp, like chianti, so that's what I called her," says Kat. Chianti, who had been let down by everyone she thought would take care of her, was cautious at first, too—like she wasn't sure she could trust Kat to stick with her. Inside the house she wouldn't let

Kat out of her sight, but when she and Kat went for walks, Chianti ran off the moment she was unleashed, triggering all Kat's insecurities and throwing her into fits of worry. Worse, at their first visit to the vet, Kat learned that her new dog had heartworms. Untreated, the vet explained, the disease could be fatal.

"I burst into tears, because I couldn't afford the treatment and I was sure she was going to die. The best I could do was to give Chianti the monthly heartworm preventative and hope it had some effect. I made her health my priority. I was like a single mother with a newborn. I stopped partying all night and took on extra hours at work to buy her organic, grain-free dog food. She often ate better than I did. And as I worked my butt off to restore her health and build a more stable life, we started to trust each other and gain self-respect, things neither of us had experienced in a long time."

When Kat was offered a higher-paying job in Brevard, North Carolina, she jumped on the opportunity to give them both a better life. In the small, charming tourist town, she and Chianti got in the habit of taking long walks after work, then sitting on the front patio of a downtown restaurant, where Kat read while Chianti greeted people. "Six months later, all these people who had started talking to Chianti had become our friends," recalls Kat.

One day, Kat's roommate brought home an additional roommate, a tall, pretty brunette with a strong spirit. Her name was Amber, and she worked in construction. Kat and Amber were attracted to each other but tried to ignore it. So Chianti took matters into her own hands. "Normally when I was at work, Chianti would just lie on my bed and do nothing—not even drink water. But she courted Amber. She'd go outside with her and play," says Kat. "I was terrified of getting close and going through the pain of losing someone. But I trusted Chianti's judgment. If she could accept Amber into the pack, I figured I should get to know her, too."

Talking to Amber, Kat discovered, felt less like getting to know a stranger than reuniting with an old friend. Ten months after they met, they stood at the top of a nearby hill in a lush, wooded glade, surrounded by a small group of friends and family, and had their first commitment ceremony. "The light was coming through the trees, and Amber and I wore dressy tops and skirts with bare feet. Chianti sat quietly beside me for part of our vows, then went to mingle with the guests and plop in the nearby creek to cool off," recalls Kat. "Life is surprising and strange. I thought I'd always live on the fringes of society and never get close to anyone. Now, here I am, eleven years later, with a wife, a job, and a stable, happy life. And I owe it all to a homeless dog who reminded me how good it feels to give and receive love."

The Ancient Alliance Between Humans and Animals

There it is again in Kat and Chianti's tale: love. It's the central theme of nearly every human-animal narrative that's ever been told—and for good reason. From the time we're born, we're students of love. We learn how to develop that deep affection through healthy bonding—with our parents, our siblings, our friends, and eventually romantic partners and spouses. Along the way, our experiences teach us how to relate to people and whom to trust—and if those interactions leave us wounded, even the toughest among us can start building walls around our hearts, or withdraw entirely, like Kat did. We no longer trust, as Buddhist teacher Jack Kornfield put it during a radio interview in San Francisco in 2005, that "our heart has the capacity to open to the sorrows as well as the beauty of the world." Love is a risk. It exposes us to potential pain and makes us vulnerable. But shutting down prevents us from moving through the healthy cycle of attachment and bonding and separation and grieving we talked about in Chapter 1. Distrusting human connection hampers our ability to fully experience life, with all its raptures and sorrows. It's a rejection, in essence, of love.

When I read Kat's Mutual Rescue submission, what drew me in was how deeply alienated she had become from the world. Bruised and wary, she had chosen to make her way alone. It was only by meeting a fellow solo traveler, who was still open to connecting despite her own history of heartbreak, that Kat was able to restore her faith in relationships.

Intrigued by the idea that animals can potentially restore people's trust in humankind, I thought of Brian Hare, an evolutionary biologist and founder of the Duke Canine Cognition Center, whom I met several years ago when he spoke at Humane Society Silicon Valley. At nineteen, Hare, with the assistance of his childhood dog, Oreo, made the breakthrough discovery that dogs understand human gestures—something scientists had always believed was an ability limited to people. That was nearly three decades ago, and he's been studying canine intelligence ever since. By now, he knows as much about dogs' minds as most of us know about our own. We reconnected with Hare to find out how pets could reach emotionally wounded people, and his response echoed what Kurt Kotrschal said: "Dog minds and human minds have both been engineered by evolution to seek out social bonds, so becoming attached is natural for both of us—and bonding with an animal offers unique advantages. They pretty much ignore your weaknesses and faults. They love you, no strings attached."

But in order to truly make sense of how a relationship with a creature of a different species can help build trust, Hare added, it helps to understand a deeper story—one that began long ago, before iPhones or cars or covered wagons or farming, back in the days when wolves roamed the landscape and humans lived by hunting and gathering. In that primitive time, an improbable friendship was born—and the story of that friendship offers crucial insight into how a chance meeting between a troubled young woman and a neglected juvenile dog was able to change both their lives.

The tale begins 35,000 years ago, says Hare, when predatory wolves began approaching human encampments to seek out a plentiful but curious (as in disgusting) source of nourishment: human poop. "Hunting prey was dangerous, even for wolves," he explains. "But ancient humans ate what wolves ate, and then left it, in a predigested, perfectly harmless form, on the ground. The smart wolves figured out it was far safer to eat poop than kill a wild animal."

This unusual turn of events changed the course of history. Only the wolves that were the least aggressive and least threatening were able to get close enough to human populations to take advantage of this safe, reliable source of food, giving those mellower beasts a leg up in the Darwinian lottery and allowing them to pass their docile DNA along to the next generation.

Humans who were tolerant of the companionable wolves got a survival boost, too. The animals were not only valuable hunting allies, availing humans of more consistent access to food, but also a reliable alarm system, with barks that could alert them to approaching danger. Over centuries, these two predators at the top of the food chain learned first to trust each other, then to rely on each other, then to love each other. Abetted by willing humans, the amicable wolves bred and thrived, their mutating genes making them ever more distinct from their fearsome ancestors, until eventually, sometime between 30,000 and 16,000 years ago, they morphed into *Canis lupus familiaris*—the Fidos and Buddys and Bellas and Dukes that 60 million Americans have in their homes and 73 percent welcome into their beds.

This new genus wasn't just friendlier, says Hare. Along with their easygoing dispositions came, for reasons scientists can't explain, a host of other changes that by happenstance are super appealing to humans. They had curly tails and cute faces, with short, wide snouts and floppy ears. Their brains had more serotonin, the chemical linked to happiness and relaxation. They acquired an uncanny knack for understanding human gestures. Emboldened, they made more eye contact, a bedrock bonding behavior. And they developed, through a happy quirk of evolution, not only a fierce devotion to us but also a unique—in my mind semi-miraculous—ability to tap into our genetic hardwiring for nurturing offspring and falling in love. When wolves evolved into dogs they essentially hacked the innate system meant to encourage us to entrust our hearts to other humans and stimulate and cement long-term bonding.

Just as wolves, in a sense, domesticated themselves, wild cats did, too—though their transformation from ferocious feline to the languid creatures that loll on our sofas is in ways even more improbable, because their ancestors were more solitary in nature. Dogs evolved from pack animals that thrived on living in close proximity to one another; long before they teamed up with us, they were social creatures who hunted together and even helped one another raise their young. Housecats, according to DNA analysis published in 2007, descend from a subspecies of cat known as *Felis silvestris lybica*. Like most wild cats, except lions, they were independent hunters, fiercely protective of their individual territory. They had to be. Felines are what is known as "obligate carnivores"—they lack certain fatty acids required to digest carbohydrates, so they eat almost nothing but protein. In the days before canned cat food filled whole shelves in grocery stores, protein was hard to come by. Ancient cats had to compete for meat not just with every other carnivore on the planet, but also with one another.

Then, about 10,000 years ago, *F. s. lybica* learned that human trash, and the mice it attracted, were easy pickings. The canniest among them weighed their options—vie with other wild predators for their precious food source or learn to get comfortable with humans—and chose us.

It didn't take long before our ancient ancestors became smitten with the beguiling felines hovering around the periphery of their dwellings. The earliest evidence suggesting that people kept cats as pets was found on the island of Cypress in the Mediterranean. Most cats are water-phobic (they can swim, but typically prefer not to), so it's unlikely they would have made their way to the island unless they came by boat—and for that they needed human assistance. But reach it they did. In a shallow grave from 9,500 years ago, a human body was found curled in an affectionate pose around an array of stone tools, a few seashells, and the bones of an eight-month-old cat.

Wolves began the slow evolutionary march toward dogdom 35,000 years ago, so in scientific terms, domestic cats are still comparatively young. Felines have changed so little since *F. s. lybica* first began prowling human trash heaps that, for years, scientists' efforts to pinpoint when they began to bond with humans were stymied because even the most archaic fossils are virtually indistinguishable from the creatures that purr for belly rubs today.

As a result, we have less knowledge about early cats. No one even knows for certain why humans were drawn to the sleek, sharp-toothed animals. One practical theory holds that cats made themselves useful by disposing of mice and snakes. But it's just as likely, other experts say, that people were won over by their sheer adorableness. In 1941, Nobel-winning Austrian zoologist and ethologist Konrad Lorenz proposed the concept known as "baby schema": that humans (and many mammals) are genetically wired to have a weakness for creatures with infant-like traits—round eyes, chubby cheeks, broad foreheads, snub noses—in order to motivate caretaking and enhance our offspring's survival. When wolves evolved into dogs, they developed some of these captivating attributes. But cats come by them naturally. It's quite possible that felines became fixtures in Egyptian homes 3,600 years ago in large part because of our innate obsession with all things cute.

Among these *awww*-inspiring creatures, the ones bold enough to come close to humans had the greatest access to food and therefore were the most likely to reproduce; as those daring cats propagated, each successive generation began edging slightly farther along the continuum from standoffish to snuggly. Once cats got comfortable enough to curl up in humans' laps, felines, like canines millennia before, became ever more affectionate and attached to us, triggering our deeply ingrained reflex to bond. And bond we did—passionately and inexorably. Today about 96 million cats are cozied up in homes across the United States. And many of them, as I've seen over and over again through the years, have, like dogs, an important thing or two to teach us about trust, bonding, and love.

Helping Traumatized Children Feel Safe and Rebuild Trust

In a manual on using animals to help children overcome a history of trauma, Debi Grebenik, PhD, a child trauma specialist in Colorado Springs, Colorado, shares the story of Mandy, an eight-year-old girl who experienced violence and abuse in her birth home. When Grebenik came across Mandy's story, the child had entered the foster care system just months before and been placed in her first home, with a family who lives on a farm. The transition was difficult. Mandy wouldn't take showers or respond to simple requests and had trouble sleeping. But a stray cat—one of the many critters on the farm—began following her everywhere.

The cat snuggled her to sleep at night and trailed after her into the bathroom, sitting with her patiently. With the feline keeping watch, Mandy eventually felt safe enough to begin showering. As the months passed, her schoolwork improved. She learned to manage her emotions more effectively. And she developed a deeper connection with her foster parents—a connection the parents attribute, in part, to the trusting relationship she built with the cat. "The family cat provided the connection she needed to begin to bond with her foster parents," Grebenik told us via email. "A strong relationship between animal and child creates a bond that can lead to healing in the child's heart."

This isn't just a one-off anecdote. Recent research at the University of Bath in the United Kingdom provides a glimpse into how deeply beneficial it can be for traumatized foster children to develop an attachment with animals. For the study, the researchers interviewed eight children between the ages of ten and sixteen who had a history of significant attachment difficulties in foster care and, as a result, had been placed in (and asked to leave) at least six different homes. One child had already been with ten different foster families in seven years. When the study began, they had all been placed in a new home within the past year. Each home had a dog. Through interviews with the children and the kids' weekly diaries, the researchers developed a real-time picture of the central role pets played in the children's lives.

The results were heartrending—and hopeful. The researchers found that kids' relationships with dogs provided comfort and solace when they were upset and bolstered their confidence to explore the world; animals served as both a safe haven and secure base, two hallmarks of healthy attachment, the vital missing ingredient they most urgently needed in their lives. In an email, Sam Carr, the study's lead author, told us that the development of secure attachment may be the single most important goal for foster children. "The bond children create with pets can serve as a bridge so they can begin to experience their foster caregivers as caring and trustworthy. Animals play an important part in helping foster children develop secure, warm, and loving relationships. Although our study focused exclusively on relationships with dogs, our anecdotal experiences and discussions with the children led us to believe that cats could be equally likely to fulfill the same functions in relation to trust, bridging, and emotional security," he explained.

In a small school with many disadvantaged students in Davenport, Iowa, Sarah McGlynn, too, has seen how a single dependable animal has the power to reach wary youngsters who have learned that adults are often unreliable—or worse. "Our students come from a very high need, high trauma, drug-affected community," says Sarah, a teacher for thirteen years. "The majority of the families live well below the poverty line. There's addiction, incarceration, and in some cases, abuse—circumstances that can seriously undermine children's peace of mind and ability to focus. These little kids are always on guard, scanning the room, waiting for the other shoe to drop."

Over the years, Sarah had brought a friend's dog into the classroom and watched in astonishment how the children responded. So when she and her boyfriend began looking for a dog to adopt nearly three years ago, they did so, in part, because Sarah wanted a therapy dog as a partner in the classroom. Their search led them to Ziggy, a half golden retriever, half German shepherd puppy. "He and his littermates—there were five boys and five girls—had been rescued from a farm," she says. "Ziggy was the alpha pup. He came running right up to me. I knew he might be harder to train than mellower dogs, but it didn't matter. We loved everything about him—and I sensed that he had the calm, steady temperament that would help my students feel safe."

At first Ziggy's behavior was challenging—he climbed over every baby gate they put in place to keep him in the kitchen, including two stacked on top of each other—but they intensified his training, and he took to it quickly. By the time he was a year old, Ziggy was a certified therapy dog.

From the day Sarah began bringing him to school with her, she saw an effect on her students. Ziggy put them at ease. Around him, the children let their guard down. "When kids sit on the floor and pet him it's almost like they go into a trance," says Sarah. Ziggy also helps them become more aware of their own behavior. "They all want to read to Ziggy or give him a treat, but he doesn't like to be around kids who are loud or bouncing off the walls," Sarah explains. "They quickly learn that in order to be around Ziggy you need to have self-control—and he rewards them by giving them a kiss or a snuggle."

More important, Ziggy gives the children who lack healthy attachments a trustworthy companion with whom they can bond. "Before students can engage academically they need to have their basic needs of safety and security met," she says. "The love that Ziggy provides helps all my trauma-affected students develop the courage to trust themselves, trust the environment of school, and trust me as their teacher."

Why We Fall So Hard for Four-Legged Creatures

By being trustworthy, Ziggy and Chianti, and the millions of cats and dogs who inhabit our homes, are able to coax wounded people out of the corners into which they've retreated. And when we begin to interact with animals, something dynamic happens: They engage our inborn drive to form attachments. At the core of that complex, unconscious attachment system is oxytocin, a hormone so potent it affects our brain and behavior as powerfully as many drugs. Sometimes called the "cuddle hormone," it has been linked to love, morality, and trust. Experts disagree about some of the particulars of oxytocin, but research is clear on its most striking effects: It not only surges in mothers and newborns during breast-feeding, but also spikes when we hold hands or hug someone and skyrockets when we have sex and fall in love. It also increases when we pet animals or look into their eyes—and dogs and cats experience a rise, too, when we interact with them, according to Paul Zak, an oxytocin researcher at Claremont Graduate University in Claremont, California, who has studied human-animal interactions. When we caught up with Zak by phone, he told us, "If love is a neurologic state marked by a rise in oxytocin, it's safe to say our animals love us."

Zak's studies have shown that when someone trusts us—and that someone can be an animal—our brains produce oxytocin, which motivates us to be both more trusting and trustworthy. At the same time, oxytocin pushes us toward people, encouraging social interaction and fostering relationships and bonding. "It actually generates a feeling of reward in the brain, so it motivates you to want to engage in future social interactions," Zak says. "As humans, we're constantly balancing a natural and appropriate fear of strangers with the rewards of being in relationships. When you have more oxytocin, the balance shifts your brain toward wanting to connect with others."

The alchemy that occurred in Sarah's classroom is likely due at least in part to oxytocin—and it's similar to what happened to Kat when she experienced Chianti's affection. By demonstrating that she was trustworthy, Chianti broke down the barriers Kat had constructed to keep people out and showed her what she was missing. "Before I met Chianti, I'd always run with an angry group of anarchists and punk rockers. With my tattoos and piercings, I look tough, too. But Chianti saw the real me, and she taught me how to do that with others—to bond with *people*, not their politics or ideals or music. She led me back into the fold of my family. I'm close with my parents now. And she helped me build a close-knit group of very loyal and trusting friends."

Animals Can Open Hearts—and Minds

While rescue pets can change the trajectory of people whose emotional development has been derailed by trauma, they can also be beneficial to the rest of us, who have healthy attachments with friends and family but still harbor blind spots or prejudice based on skin color, say, or net worth, religion, or sexual orientation. It can even open your eyes to different *species*. It's common for people to define themselves as a "cat person" or a "dog person," as if you have to be one or the other. But that kind of thinking can limit your capacity for happiness, as I learned when I was a child and witnessed for the first time the mysterious power pets have to cut through people's preconceived notions and open their hearts.

My father, Fred, was many things: the son of Italian immigrants, an award-winning chemist, an aficionado of snapdragons and sunflowers, an inveterate whistler, and for me, far younger than my two older siblings, a source of wisdom, sounding board, and encourager-in-chief. The one thing he wasn't: a cat lover. "Carol, don't kiss the cat," he'd admonish me over and over. "Cats have germs." *Germs?* Cats had slinky grace, satiny fur, lullaby-like purrs, whiskers that tickled. I adored them—and since my mother did, too, our family was never without a feline or two. Her love of animals was (and is) one of the few things she and I shared—and her appreciation only made my father's aversion that much more unfathomable. My dad was my mainstay. I wanted him to share my joy. How could I help him understand the satisfaction and pleasure of loving a cat?

The answer was simple: I couldn't. But Chester could. He arrived in our home in 1976, when I was eleven. A husky orange tabby with tigerish stripes and a face that looked like someone had dribbled white paint from the tip of his nose down each of his cheeks, Chester belonged to my older sister's friends. Their landlord had discovered they had a cat and given them an ultimatum: relinquish the animal or the lease. While they scrambled to look for new housing, Chester came to live with us. My father wasn't pleased. We already had Lucinda, a needy feline with black fur, whom my mom and I adored and my father ignored. But Chester, we soon learned, was Lucinda's opposite—and not just physically.

When my parents had parties, Lucinda hid while Chester would sprawl on the floor in the middle of the festivities, savoring the revelry. He was a total ham. But the purest difference went deeper: When Lucinda jumped on your lap she wanted love—and I was only too happy to provide it; when Chester did, he wanted to *give* you love. He'd tilt his head back and stare into your eyes. He craved *connection*. With everyone.

Dad was a man of habit, and every Friday night at eight p.m. he migrated to the den, where he'd kick back in his orange leather chair and watch PBS's *Wall Street Week* with Louis Rukeyser. Mom and I had no interest in the show—but Chester did. On a Friday night soon after he came to live with us, he followed my dad upstairs, jumped into his lap, and burrowed into the crook of his arm to watch, too. The next Friday he did the same. And the Friday after that. Several months after Chester came to stay with us, my sister announced that her friends were ready to take their cat back. My dad looked stricken. "Tell them we'd like to keep him," he said. And that was that. Chester became a fixture, not just in our family's life but in my dad's.

I was delighted—and puzzled. What magic did Chester possess that allowed him, in the course of a few months, to completely capture my father's heart? It so stumped me that I thought about it periodically over the years. One day, while sitting home in a particularly lonely period of my life, I was again mulling Chester's ability to break through my dad's resistance, and the description that popped into my mind was "open-hearted." Like Chianti, Chester, at his core, had a heart that was open to everyone—those who loved him and those who didn't—and because he loved everyone, he found love in the least likely places, including my father's arms.

Our delightful, extroverted cat lived with us for eleven years—and refused to leave my dad's side the night he died of cancer in 1986, holding vigil as resolutely as any longtime companion. By then, they'd shared a lot—me leaving for college, my dad's retirement, his grueling cancer treatments. One evening before he got sick I walked past the open door to the den and saw him looking down at Chester, lips pressed to his funny, paint-splattered mug. "Germs, huh?" I said with a smile. Dad just winked. By then, we both knew the truth. The only thing contagious about Chester—or any animal that beguiles their way into your heart—was his remarkable capacity for love.

Most companion animals possess that remarkable capacity—and *we do, too.* It's easy to forget that sometimes. But becoming attached to an animal, as Kat discovered, can help us tap into our vast ability to love and embrace the messy, challenging, fulfilling, and rewarding world of human relationships, where, along with pain, we can also find genuine joy.

Kat says Chianti is slowing down these days. More white hair is sprinkled in with her dark coat, and her easy, loping gait has grown stiff and slow. "She goes outside more often at night and gazes up at the stars, like she's contacting her home planet," says Kat. "She's been a fine dog and a dear companion—better than I could have asked for and possibly better than I deserved. All those years when I took her for walks, I thought I was in charge. I was wrong. She was the one leading me—back to safety, back to stability, back to love. She found me in a bar—a messed-up human headed for an early grave—and led me back to life."

3

Coping with Grief

Fur as a Source of Comfort and Solace

In February 2014, Kylie Myers, who had just turned twelve, started complaining of knee pain. The pediatrician couldn't find anything wrong—but when the pain didn't go away by late March, her mom, Robin, asked the doctor for an MRI. The results brought the Atlanta family's normal, happy life to a startling halt. Kylie had Ewing's sarcoma, a rare type of cancerous tumor that grows in the bones and nearby cartilage. It affects about two hundred children in the United States every year. "The cancer had already metastasized, so it was very serious. We were shocked and frightened. But we were hopeful that, with chemotherapy and radiation, she'd be able to fight the disease."

If anyone could beat cancer, Robin and her husband, Mark, told themselves, Kylie could. From the moment she was born, Smiley Kylie, as they called her, astonished her parents and three older sisters with her exuberance and mischievous wit. "She just had this gift for joy," says Mark. "In school, Kylie was the first one to welcome the new kid, she was a peacemaker among her three older sisters, she sang all the time and was crazy about Broadway musicals. She loved making people smile." When her school put on the play *Annie*, nine-year-old Kylie was cast in the lead. The role's showstopping lyrics, "The sun will come out tomorrow," suited her. Kylie didn't just sing those words. She believed them.

The rigors of chemo, however, strained even her sunny outlook. Over the ensuing ten months, Kylie lost her hair, along with 30 percent of her body weight. Sores lined her mouth and esophagus, making it too painful to eat. She contracted *C. difficile*, a violent, difficult-to-treat gastrointestinal infection. Her parents had to feed her through a tube in her stomach every thirty minutes to make sure she took in enough calories.

"It was brutal, but Kylie fought for moments of joy—like when she painted her bald head orange for Halloween and when, during a stay in the hospital near Christmastime, she asked a nurse if she could stick a medical instrument up my nose to see if it would glow like Rudolph," says Mark. But what Kylie really wanted, as she told her parents repeatedly, was a kitten. She brought it up not long after her diagnosis, and by January, when she started radiation—the nine-week treatment they were hoping would drive the cancer into remission—she began pestering them. "We already had two dogs and two cats—all rescues—and we were driving to Charlotte five days a week for radiation, so we told her, 'Let's finish radiation and then we'll see,'" recalls Robin.

On the final day of radiation, the moment they'd been looking forward to for ten months, Kylie said her shoulder hurt. Her doctor ordered a scan. It revealed that the cancer had spread throughout her body. There was nothing more the doctors could do.

Stunned, the Myerses bundled up their daughter, wheeled her to the car, and drove her home. Mark carried her into the house, like he'd done dozens of times over the past ten months. By then, she felt like a life-size doll in his arms. "She looked up at him with her huge eyes and said, '*Now* can I have that baby kitty?'" recalls Robin.

Mark called a friend who was involved with Angels Among Us, a local animal rescue organization. "Within an hour, they brought us this ten-week-old tortoiseshell kitten with yellow eyes—Kylie's favorite color," he says. "When the rescue group received the kitten, she was malnourished and ill, and when they brought her to us she'd just been treated for fleas. The little bugs were still literally falling off her. One eye was matted from the medication they were using to treat her ulcerated cornea. Her fur was all scraggly. But Kylie didn't care. That kitty was the answer to her prayers."

When her parents put the tiny feline in their daughter's spindly arms, Kylie beamed her trademark smile and announced, "Her name is Eliza but you shall call her Liza."

Robin and Mark will never forget that smile. It was the last one their dimpled daughter was able to muster.

"It was such a gift to see her joy at getting the one last thing she wanted," recalls Robin. "Liza curled up against Kylie's body and wrapped her paw around her arm, as if she knew her mission was to love on Kylie." And there the kitten stayed, getting off Kylie's bed only to use the litter box, for two days, until the Myerses' youngest daughter took her final breath and let go.

In the boggy, quicksand months that followed, the family was overwhelmed by a sadness they never knew was possible. "I couldn't eat or sleep. I could barely speak in complete sentences. I was fully aware that my world had changed forever—that I would never again experience total, unalloyed joy and that I would never have all my children together with me in this lifetime," says Robin. "My grief felt like a physical crushing weight, and heaviness permeated my body."

Before she passed, Kylie told Mark that she wanted him to find a cure for childhood cancer. She looked at Robin and said, "Take care of my baby kitten." As they tried to adjust to the unimaginable, the bereft couple used Kylie's parting words as instructions for how to move forward. As Mark set about looking for work in a cancer-related field, Robin poured her love and energy into caring for Liza.

The kitten made her task easy. "She was content to sit in my lap and cuddle most of the day, and I carried her with me everywhere, almost unconsciously. Taking care of Liza was one of the few things on which I was able to focus, because it felt like I was still doing something for Kylie," she says. "Liza seemed to want to offer me love and comfort. If she wasn't right there when I started to cry, she'd come from wherever she was in the house and curl up in my lap. I've never had an animal who seemed so attuned to what I needed. She's always willing to share my grief, quietly and tenderly. She takes me in whatever frame of mind I'm in."

For all her snuggliness, Liza is also a playful cat, and her antics make the family laugh, much as Kylie did while she was alive. "When I'm with Liza I feel Kylie's presence—her joy, her silliness, her love. We all do, and that has been a blessing for our other daughters as well. Liza is a beautiful reminder of their much-adored baby sister," says Robin. "Every time Liza does something funny, like insisting on burrowing under the blanket on my lap when I'm watching TV, I think, 'Kylie would love this.' I'm so incredibly grateful to the people who rescued Liza—not only because they made her available for Kylie, but because she's been such a blessing for me. I think Kylie knew that was going to happen. She was a smart, intuitive little girl, wise beyond her years. When Kylie told me to take care of Liza, I think she also whispered to Liza to take care of me. She knew her kitty's mission wasn't over. It had really just begun."

Sharing Kylie and Liza's Message of Hope

Not long after we put out a call for Mutual Rescue stories, Mark sent a note about their family's experience. In it he wrote, "There is no pain greater than that of losing a child. Sometimes the pain is so great that I don't know how we keep moving. But this I know: We couldn't have budged without Liza." It was among the most wrenching submissions I'd read, and we decided to reach out to the Myerses to ask if we could feature their extraordinary story in our second Mutual Rescue film.

When Robin and Mark agreed, I experienced a pang of worry. Their trust felt sacred—like I'd been handed a priceless, one-of-a-kind vase. We had an obligation to honor their experience.

If the response to the film, which shared Robin and Mark's moving, honest account of their ordeal, is any indication, we succeeded.

The Mutual Rescue film *Kylie & Liza* has been viewed 12.6 million times since its launch. But it was the outpouring of insightful comments that I found particularly touching. "Miracles come to us in all sorts of shapes and forms, even in a tiny kitten," said one post. "Some angels choose whiskers and fur over wings and a halo," said another. "Cats are intuitive, and they know when you need them," wrote a third. Then there was this: "We are all connected. The power of us realizing and accepting this is overwhelming. Love creates the most powerful bridges."

Kylie and Liza's story reveals that we can endure even the most terrible losses. At its heart, it's a film about hope. The Myerses' sadness won't ever go away. They miss their daughter every day. But the love between the Myers family and Liza did indeed create a bridge—one that was strong enough to span even the fathomless abyss of grief.

A New Look at Weathering Grief

If bonding with a person or animal is the exhilarating part of the attachment cycle, grief is its unbearable side—the yin to love's yang, the agony to its ecstasy. But the light and dark of attachment are as inextricably linked as day and night. In *A Grief Observed*, writer C. S. Lewis's collection of reflections following the death of his wife, he says, "Bereavement is an integral and universal part of our experience of love. It is not the truncation of the process but one of its phases; not the interruption of the dance, but the next figure." Katherine Shear, MD, a leading grief researcher and professor of psychiatry at Columbia University School of Social Work, puts it more succinctly: "Grief is a form of love."

No one who experiences the joy of attachment escapes the ache of loss. Every year approximately 2.5 million people in the United States die, leaving behind, on average, four close bereaved friends and family members. And that's not counting all the millions of beloved pets that, when they pass, leave a tender cat- or dog-shaped void in our lives—or the many other sources of grief, due to divorce, job loss, fractured friendships, or even the happy-sad occasion of children leaving home for college, that befall many of us throughout our lives.

Yet, for an experience that's so universal, most of us know surprisingly little about bereavement, save for a vague awareness, left over from Psych 101, of the five stages of grief—denial, anger, bargaining, depression, and acceptance—that psychiatrist Elisabeth Kübler-Ross laid out in the late sixties. As a culture, we're uncomfortable with death and dying, so we've paid little attention to what grief feels like, how people heal, or what helps them knit together the raw edges of the wound. There's no way to truly prepare ourselves for the many losses we all face, much less the loss of someone we adore, but our lack of understanding leaves us painfully ill-equipped to handle mourning—and makes the impact of tragedy that much harder to bear.

Now, science is beginning to shed more light on grieving. Since the 1960s, studies have expanded on Kübler-Ross's groundbreaking work to reveal that, while many bereaved people experience those five emotions, the path of anguish is rarely so tidy. Instead, it seems to follow a stumbling two-steps-forward-one-step-back pattern that's as individual, fluid, and unpredictable as loss itself, and often spans, in no particular order, a variety of emotions and stages. Shock. Disbelief. Denial. Yearning and searching for the deceased. Numbness. Withdrawal. Guilt. Disorganization. Anger. Despair.

The shape bereavement takes varies depending on who (or what) you lost and how you lost them; it cuts deeper and can be more difficult to process when a death is sudden, when someone you love takes their own life, or when you lose a child or the person (or animal) you love the most in the world. Some losses leave wounds so deep it's hard to imagine they will ever heal.

But even in the most shattering circumstances, we can reorient ourselves toward joy by facing and dealing with the pain. For many, friends and family help; others rely on trained therapists to guide them toward a place of acceptance. And those of us with companion animals may, like Robin Myers, find their unwavering support and comfort to be a safe haven, in the parlance of attachment theory—a touchstone that grounds us and helps us find our way through the fog. When Swedish researchers conducted in-depth interviews with twelve adult patients who were dying and receiving palliative care in their homes, as well as their grieving family members, they discovered that a significant number turned to their pets when they felt insecure and vulnerable. Participants who had cats or dogs said their animals' attention, their joy, and their avid interest in being around their owners even when they were sad or exhausted had a meaningful effect on their sense of peace and security.

The Many Ways Pets Support Us Through Sorrow

The Swedish study of patients in palliative care hints at why animals can be such powerful medicine for the bereaved, but I sensed there had to be more to it. To find out, we called Cori Bussolari, PsyD, associate professor in the department of counseling psychology at the University of San Francisco, who has researched coping and bereavement and runs support groups for people who are grieving the loss of a pet. "On the most basic level, animals force people to maintain a routine," she explains. "Get out of bed. Feed the cat. Walk the dog. Clean the litter box. It forces them to stay engaged."

Beyond that practical aspect lies a host of emotional benefits. While research shows that one of the most potent coping mechanisms for grief is the support we receive from other people, says Bussolari, humans can be unpredictable and don't always respond the way we want or need them to. People may say well-intentioned things that feel completely wrong to someone who is grieving, like, "He's in a better place" or "It was her time."

"Animals never say the wrong thing," says Bussolari.

Likewise, grieving people often worry about how they'll be perceived. They might think, *If I'm crying am I going to push friends away or make them uncomfortable?* With cats and dogs, you don't have to worry that they're judging you. As Robin says, "My family and dear friends accept me where I am and are so kind and supportive, but I don't want to be a dark cloud to everyone wherever I go. When Liza offers me love and comfort, I don't have to worry that I'm sucking the joy from everyone around me. I don't make her life harder when I'm falling apart. There is comfort in that, and there's comfort in the fact that Liza has no expectations for how I should be doing."

Dogs and cats can also be helpful because they're often acutely—sometimes uniquely—tuned in to our suffering. Several years ago, researchers at the University of London recruited eighteen dog owners, along with their canines—twelve of whom were adopted from a rescue facility—to participate in an experiment designed to test empathy, or at least empathy-like responding, in animals. For the experiment, the dog's owner and a stranger whom the dog had never met sat and talked for two minutes while the canine was in the room. Then the humans took turns pretending to either cry (with their face in their hands) or hum "Mary Had a Little Lamb" for twenty seconds each. The animals' responses were extraordinary. Nearly all the dogs came over to nuzzle or lick the crying person, regardless of whether it was their owner or a total stranger, while they paid little attention to either person when they were humming or talking. "The majority of the dogs behaved in a manner that was consistent with empathic concern and comfort-offering," the researchers concluded.

As comforting, animals' empathy has no time limit. They don't become impatient if sadness lingers, as it often does after the death of a cherished loved one. "Friends and family usually do a great job of supporting a bereaved person for a month or two, but then they get busy and expect life to go back to normal. A cat or dog may be the only creature in your life that is there once the initial outpouring of support dies down—and they won't tell you to buck up if you're still crying a year, or ten years, after the loss," says Bussolari.

Pets' steadfastness can be crucial, since grief isn't something you get over in a few weeks, like the flu. Even those who regain their footing relatively quickly may be struck by pangs of longing and sadness for years. Indeed, one of the central challenges of grief—learning to love someone in their absence—is also its most heartbreaking. As Thomas Attig, past president of the Association for Death Education and Counseling, says in his book *The Heart of Grief*, "Grieving is a journey that teaches us how to love in a new way now that our loved one is no longer with us." Death ends a life, but it doesn't end a relationship, or love.

As mourners search for ways to maintain a relationship with those they've lost and continue loving and honoring their memories, pets can be a conduit for continued connection, by providing a tangible link to the past and, often, a meaningful association with the person who is gone. As vital, points out Bussolari, cats and dogs allow us—sometimes *force* us—to take mini breaks from our grief. When Robin is watching TV and Liza burrows under the blanket on her lap, making her laugh, the cat lifts the pall of Robin's sadness—and those simple, fleeting glimpses of normalcy can be the breadcrumbs that eventually lead the sick-at-heart back to a place where the loss still hurts but no longer consumes them or obliterates their ability to function.

The Palliative Power of a One-Eyed Cat

After Mindy Beeler's mom took her own life in March 2015, Mindy's body felt so weighted with sorrow she could barely get out of bed, and she was too nauseated to eat. "My mom was my best friend, my confidante, my strongest supporter," says Mindy, thirty-six, of Louisville, Kentucky. "She had me when she was only fourteen, so we sort of grew up together. We understood each other. We both adored animals. We both had rheumatoid arthritis, and like her I've struggled with depression. But I couldn't believe she'd leave us. I couldn't believe our family wasn't enough to make her want to stay."

The lone bright spot in her life was her cat, Dorian. Mindy had taken Dorian and his five siblings in as ailing kittens. "Dorian was the puniest of all and had a terrible eye infection that required ointment every two hours around the clock," she says. "He lost his eye, but he didn't seem to mind. He was hilarious and playful. I found good homes for the other kittens, but I couldn't bear to part with him."

One morning several months after her mom died, Mindy woke up crying. "I missed my mom so much and wanted more than anything to talk to her. I just kept thinking, 'What's the point? Why do I care whether I live or not?' I had a gun in my closet and started thinking about how easy it would be to use it," she says. "Then Dorian came and stood over me and meowed right in my face, staring at me with his one eye. He swatted gently at my face, inviting me to play. In spite of the terrible ache in my heart, I started laughing. I couldn't help it. He's just so darn funny. In that moment I realized I wasn't going to use the gun. I was going to keep going, not just for myself, but for him. My mom loved hearing stories about Dorian. I think she knew he was the angel who would help me cope after she was gone."

Furry Solace in Funeral Homes

Many types of animals can ease the anguish of grief, but dogs' ability to soothe the bereaved is becoming so well accepted that increasing numbers of funeral homes are bringing canines onto the staff, according to the National Funeral Directors Association. In February 2014, Doug Wagemann, co-owner of several funeral homes in California, unexpectedly found himself one of them.

Doug was meeting with a family whose elderly parents had died within several days of each other, when they asked if they could bring their parents' orphaned teacup poodle, Lady, into the funeral home. "In the middle of the meeting, I felt some light scratches on my thigh," Doug recalls. "The tiny dog was standing on her hind legs and shaking like a leaf, so I reached down, picked her up and held her in my lap, where she put her head on my arm and fell asleep. A feeling of intense compassion came over me. I've had pets in the past but I'd never experienced anything like this in my sixty-three years. This poor little creature had lost both her people within a few days. She was obviously grieving and afraid, and my heart just went out to her."

When the meeting was over, Doug asked what the family's plans were for Lady. "They told me they were going to try to find a home for her, but if they couldn't they were considering putting her down," recalls Doug. "I said, 'I'm not looking for a dog, but before you make any major decisions, please give me a call.'"

Several days later, they did. "They said they wanted me to have her," he says. "She's been our little princess ever since."

For the prior two years, as her former owners' health deteriorated, Lady had been kept in a crate and was only let out to eat and relieve herself—and even then she went on newspaper inside. "When I adopted her, I looked her square in the eye and promised, 'I'm going to give you as much life experience as possible for the time you have left,'" he says. "She comes to work with me every day, and through meeting our clients, she has found a new purpose. I've seen Lady be the conduit for conversations among siblings who haven't spoken to each other in years. I've seen her ease kids' stress and normalize the experience of being at a funeral home. I've seen her help people with Alzheimer's come out of their fog and begin to understand what we're talking about. I've seen a two-hundred-fifty-pound diesel truck mechanic reach out to hold her to help him through his sadness."

Adopting a small, older dog has enriched Doug's life as well. "She has reduced my stress and forced me to get out and walk more. And she reminds me what's important. Lady gives love so freely and selflessly. She has influenced so many lives, but she's not egotistical. She's not proud. There's a lesson in there for all of us."

One urgent lesson from Lady's story is that, while older animals are less likely to be adopted, we not only do them a grim disservice by overlooking their promise, but we also curtail our own opportunities for growth and joy. Imagine what would have been lost if Lady had been put down! She wouldn't have had the chance to realize her full potential, and hundreds of people's lives, including Doug's, would have been a bit darker, their burdens a bit heavier, without the blessing of her presence.

I Know the Sorrow of Losing a Companion Animal

When I was living in my lonely house in Santa Rosa and running a company for Intuit, my two cats, Wiley and Wilbur, were my family. Like every family, our lives were enmeshed. We had a daily routine. We took care of one another. We needed one another, entertained one another, periodically annoyed one another, unfailingly adored one another. When Wilbur started losing weight and acting sluggish, I was concerned, but not alarmed. He was only ten—not worryingly old for a feline. Nevertheless, I took him to the vet, where he was, to my horror, diagnosed with cancer.

We tried several treatments. Each bought my dear boy a little time, but eventually the day came when his suffering was unbearable and it was time to say goodbye. Letting go of Wilbur felt like cutting off a limb. I'd never met a cat that was funnier than Wilbur, and few could top his kind heart. After a long day of work, I'd often collapse on the sofa, not just tired but numb, like icicles had grown around my heart. I'd drape my arm over the back cushion, and Wilbur would pour himself into the crook of my arm and purr. *And purr.* Was he doing it to help me? My brain tells me there's no way to know; my heart tells me he was. Either way, I could feel the icicles begin to melt.

I was heartbroken by Wilbur's loss. Anyone who's been there knows how devastating it is to say goodbye to an animal, but I wasn't prepared for how alone I felt. I found it difficult to talk about the loss, because some people don't understand the pain of losing a pet. Cori Bussolari says that feeling is all too common. She and other experts call pet loss "disenfranchised grief." "It's easy to feel lonely and disregarded when a companion animal dies," she says. "In our support groups for people who've lost pets, participants are relieved to realize their feelings are normal. The recognition they're not alone is often the turning point that helps them begin to make peace with the loss and move on."

I began to realize that losing my one-of-a-kind cat had opened an older, long-buried wound—the loss of my father, who had succumbed to cancer seventeen years before. If my mom was the source of my love of animals, my dad bequeathed me everything else, from my work ethic and drive to succeed and achieve to my craving for eggplant parmigiana. After he passed, I tried to ignore the deep ache in my soul by doing things that would have made him proud: working long hours and climbing the corporate ladder. But my attempt to honor him had also been a way to avoid facing the terrible pain of his loss. Now, as I mourned Wilbur's passing, I was paying the price. The depth of my sorrow was inescapable.

Wiley, my other cat, was bereft, too. He and Wilbur were best friends. He had always been happy and well-adjusted, but after Wilbur passed he followed me around the house looking lost and adrift—a common symptom of grief in animals, according to recent studies, which have shown that many types of animals mourn the loss of companions of their own species as well as others. Every time I sat down Wiley leaped onto my lap, desperate for the solace of physical contact. As we comforted each other, I slowly started to pick up the pieces of my life and move forward. Wiley was my safe haven, and I was his. The refuge we gave each other during that sad time carried us both through.

Wilbur's death forced me to see a deeper truth: The pain of loss is as integral to the process of bonding and attachment as love itself. It's all part of the natural cycle, and unless we allow ourselves to fully experience the deep, seemingly bottomless ache of grief, we won't be able to open ourselves to the full joy of new attachments.

My grief also forced me take a critical look at my life. Ever since my father died, I'd buried myself in work, isolating myself so I didn't have to risk the pain of becoming attached again. After Wilbur passed, I started thinking about my next chapter, and almost two years to the day later, I left Intuit—the career that had marked the culmination of my business-school ambitions—in search of new, even more meaningful opportunities.

Most of us are more resilient than we believe we will be when faced with the death of a cherished one, and pets can bolster our ability to cope and find renewed purpose. As writer Anne Lamott points out, "You will lose someone you can't live without, and your heart will be badly broken, and the bad news is that you never completely get over the loss of your beloved. But this is also the good news. They live forever in your broken heart that doesn't seal back up. And you come through."

Our rescue animals can play an integral role in helping us come through. Caring for Liza is one of the factors that helps Robin find meaning and feel connected to Kylie. "Living with grief has been about learning to live with terrible pain and joy intermingled. There will never be one without the other. Kylie taught us to fight for moments of joy—joy *in spite* of what we're going through. That's what she did as she battled cancer, and that's what we do to this day. Liza's spirit of joy is part of what sustains us. She's part of Kylie's legacy."

Grief is not the end of the story. If we face it and allow ourselves to experience the pain, which animals can help us feel safe enough to do, we have the opportunity to carry the memory of our dear ones forward and let their love—and the love of our animals—help us begin to write the next chapter.

4

Flourishing after Sorrow

Four-Legged Support for Post-Traumatic Growth

Jessi Burns, thirty-three, met John while they were both in grad school in Los Angeles, and she was wowed by him from the beginning. "He was getting his PhD in psychology, he played the guitar, he was this genuine, personable, well-liked guy. I was thrilled when he asked me out," she recalls. Before long, they moved in together and began talking about getting married. "We were planning our life together—talking about having kids, where we wanted to live, getting a dog. We were so in love. It was a wonderful time."

One Sunday morning when they'd been together for almost three years, Jessi woke up and found a note from John saying he'd gone to school to get some work done. She texted him. No response. She called him. No answer. Hours later, when she finally reached him, what he told her made her blood run cold: He was considering taking his own life. "I knew he was stressed out with school but I had no idea it was that bad. I thought John was a happy, well-adjusted guy. The idea that he was suicidal was *completely* shocking," she says. "I called the police, and he ended up being put in the hospital on a psychiatric hold."

John confessed to Jessi that he'd been suffering silently with depression for years. He'd never told a soul what he was going through, nor had he ever sought help. "He seemed relieved that people finally knew, and he said he was committed to getting better," she recalls.

To get back on his feet, John decided to temporarily move to his parents' house on the East Coast, where he could devote himself full-time to his emotional recovery. "It was wrenching to have him so far away, and I felt helpless because I wasn't there to support him in person," Jessi says. "When we talked on the phone he sounded like he was doing well, but phone conversations only reveal so much. I worried about him constantly."

On November 14, 2011, Jessi received the phone call that split her life in two. It was her father, who lived in Colorado and had just gotten off the phone with John's parents. John had gone through with it. He had taken his own life. "I don't remember anything about those first couple of weeks, except that I flew to Colorado Springs to be with my parents," she says. "My brain wouldn't function. I simply couldn't comprehend what had happened."

With John gone, Jessi was lost. "I couldn't get out of bed, I couldn't eat, I couldn't sleep," she says. "I felt such a sense of guilt and sadness and confusion. I asked myself over and over again what happened, and why couldn't I stop it? The person I loved the most was gone, my future was gone, and I honestly felt like I couldn't bear it. I'd never been depressed before, but I started having serious thoughts of suicide, too. It didn't feel like there was anything left to live for."

Jessi's ability to focus was so fractured she couldn't follow the plot of a TV show, much less read a book. But one day she opened her computer and, without really thinking about what she was doing, she went online and began looking at rescue dogs. "John and I had often talked about adopting a dog, so it almost felt like he was there with me—like we were still making plans and still connected," Jessi says. "I was in no shape to take care of a dog, but I knew my parents would help me—and after everything that had happened, my heart told me this was the right thing to do. As I scrolled through pictures, it was the first time I felt even a glimmer of hope."

On the website of Humane Society of the Pikes Peak Region, she saw a picture of a skinny, eight-month-old yellow Lab mix with big brown eyes staring straight into the camera. "She looked completely pitiful—sad, scared, overwhelmed. I doubt anyone else looking at that photo would have been drawn to her. But I felt an instant sense of kinship. She looked how I felt inside," says Jessi. "My dad and I went to meet her. She was underweight and had kennel cough. She was wild-eyed and skittish. I fell completely in love with her. It was the first time I thought about something other than myself and what I had lost and started imagining that I might have some other kind of future."

The dog had been found wandering in a neighborhood a week before. Despite their efforts, no one could uncover any details about her history. She wasn't spayed or chipped or wearing a collar. The pup wasn't even house-trained, as Jessi discovered once she brought her home, nor did she know how to walk on a leash. Jessi named the dog Andromeda—Andi for short—and set her mind to training and caring for the undisciplined stray. But Jessi quickly learned that the dog would be training her, too.

"Andi wouldn't let me sleep in. She'd come to the side of my bed, sit up on her haunches, and put her paws on the mattress. She always had a toy in her mouth, and she would just stare at me until I opened my eyes and got up," says Jessi. "She forced me to rejoin the world. I had to feed her and train her and walk her. On our strolls, I started talking to more people, and that made me feel well enough to start reaching out to friends."

Andi's presence also shielded Jessi from the darkness in her head. "Instead of going over and over the details of John's death and asking myself why he did it, I focused on Andi and what she needed," says Jessi. "At first it felt like a success if I could go five minutes without thinking about what happened. Then I got to the point where I could go ten minutes, or fifteen. I was still dangerously depressed. But Andi is such a playful, lovable dog. She showed me that you can find joy in the smallest things. When I pulled her leash out, it was the *best moment ever*—every single time. She taught me to be more like that—to look for small things to be happy about, whether it was a sunny day or a good conversation with a friend. Andi must have been through a lot before she was brought to the shelter, and yet she was able to move on and be happy. Eventually, I started to feel like I was inching back toward a more normal place, too."

Nine months after John died, Jessi got a job with a nonprofit in Denver that delivers meals to people with debilitating illnesses. Several years later she met a man online. "I was wary of getting into a new relationship, but Matt is wonderful. He knows everything I went through and is supportive and loving and kind. He and I adopted a second dog, Winston, from Foothills Animal Shelter, where I'd been working. Winston is Andi's best friend and has brought out the puppy in her, which has been fun to watch. Andi and I both had to start from scratch. We both had to create a new future. But because we had each other, we both learned that even when things look hopeless, there's always an opportunity for second chances."

Animals Can Help Us Bounce Back—and Sometimes Bounce Forward

I first learned about Jessi and Andi when we put out a call for Mutual Rescue stories. Hearing about their extraordinary journey from trauma and heartbreak to passion and joy left me speechless. How could such devastating circumstances end up being so redemptive and hopeful? It struck me as a true tribute to the resilience of the human spirit as well as the restorative impact of the human-animal bond. When we decided to write a book about mutual rescue experiences, their story leaped to mind—and I knew that I wanted Jessi and Andi to be part of it.

Jessi's blow was worse than most of us can imagine and more devastating than most of us will ever face. But the reality is, even far smaller losses can leave us reeling. Anything from job loss to divorce to a house fire or flood can make us feel as if we've lost our bearings, pitching even the most carefully plotted lives into disarray. And we're often left to cope with such setbacks on our own.

Our work, our relationships, our plans, and our dreams are crucial pieces of our identity, and when they suddenly disappear, it's easy to feel like we've lost part of ourselves or no longer feel certain of who we are or where we fit in the world. We lose our ability to trust ourselves, others—and sometimes even life itself. In that vulnerable, broken state we often do exactly what Jessi did: We withdraw from social activities and human contact, turning our backs on two mainstays of healthy coping—social support and staying active—that can help pull us through.

Without a secure relationship to anchor us, we're left alone with nothing to distract us from our own sadness, and it's easy to tell ourselves stories that can cause more emotional damage. *I'm a failure. No one will ever love me. I'll never find another job/partner/house/life.* As Buddhist teacher Pema Chödrön explains, "It's not what happens to us that causes us to suffer; it's how we *relate* to the things that happen to us that causes us to suffer." By dwelling on the negative, we become, in a sense, the architects of our own destruction.

And that's where rescue pets come in. Andi didn't instantly banish Jessi's suffering. But Andi's companionship gently nudged the negative narrative that had been playing in Jessi's mind in a more positive direction. Moreover, adopting a shelter animal was a courageous and hopeful act and an investment in her future—a future that wasn't going to look anything like the one she'd been dreaming about, building, and working toward. It was her way of saying, *I don't know what's going to happen, but whatever it is, I won't be alone.* It was an act of faith.

By bringing Andi into her life, relying on the dog as her secure attachment, entrusting Andi with her still-broken heart, Jessi—who had experienced loss, grief, and suffering—became not just whole again but *better* than whole. And so, it appears, did Andi.

Their story provides proof of a hopeful phenomenon: When

individuals blindly grope their way through their misery, they often discover something in themselves that allows them to rise. In the psychological realm, it's called post-traumatic growth—an uplifting, and surprisingly common, response to emotional or physical trauma. It's not that they don't suffer. Like everyone else who endures trauma, people who experience post-traumatic growth are often handicapped by pain. Trauma shatters our worldview and upends the natural order of things, forcing us to question whom and what we trust and have always believed to be true. It's at least temporarily disabling for nearly everyone.

But research shows that the long-term response to trauma varies widely. A small percentage of people are, understandably, tortured by lingering symptoms, like anxiety and nightmares, that are characteristic of post-traumatic stress disorder. (We'll explore this difficult-to-treat condition, which shows hopeful signs of responding to animal-assisted therapy, in Chapter 10.) Others gradually begin to reintegrate into the usual warp and weft of their lives and return to normal—no better or worse than they were before. But the latest research shows that at least half of people who withstand harrowing ordeals—including many who suffer from PTSD—come out of the experience with life-altering lessons or insights. "Through their misfortune, they find a deeper meaning in life, or a greater appreciation for friends and family, or a heightened sense of purpose," explains Jack Tsai, PhD, a post-traumatic growth researcher and director of the Yale School of Medicine's Division of Mental Health Services and Treatment Outcomes Research. "They often experience horrible suffering, but through that suffering they change in ways that allow them to grow."

In a sense, we all know this happens. It was Friedrich Nietzsche, a philosopher not known for his sunny optimism, who said, "That which does not kill us makes us stronger." But emotional strength is only part of the equation. With post-traumatic growth, a person who has faced difficult challenges doesn't just return to baseline. They change in fundamental, sometimes dramatic, ways—and in some cases, an animal can be the fulcrum that lifts them out of their pain. Having a loyal cat or dog doesn't guarantee that you'll thrive after trauma, nor is an animal companion a requirement for flourishing after loss. But an ally with four legs can help guide lost, ailing souls back into the rich current of life and may even, as happened with Jessi, goad them to become happier, more engaged and fulfilled than they were before.

Of course, it raises the question: *Why* do these remarkable outcomes occur? Why was Jessi able to bounce back after adopting Andi? How did a traumatized woman and a stray dog, neither of whom were functioning well on their own, begin to flourish once they found each other?

Part of the explanation has to do with the power of attachment, which we've talked about in previous chapters. Once Jessi adopted and bonded with Andi, the canine became an attachment figure. Andi was Jessi's safe haven, infusing her life with a sense of comfort and security, and her secure base, giving her the confidence to venture back into the world and try new things—and Jessi was Andi's. As their relationship blossomed, their mutual affection completed the arc of the bonding cycle we've been talking about in the last few chapters, from attachment to loss and back to love again—and carried with it the benefits of every close friendship. Together, they discovered new activities, took more risks, and had more fun.

They engaged, as psychologists say, in "active coping"—a primary contributor to post-traumatic growth. "All Andi wanted to do was play and hike and be outside, so she pulled me into that realm, too," Jessi says. "We spent a lot of time alone together, and she's such a joyful dog she started to make me happy, too—and that helped me take concrete steps to confront my grief. I joined Survivors of Suicide support groups, and found it was incredibly helpful to talk to people who understood exactly what I was going through. No one likes to talk about suicide. Once I joined the support groups, I learned how incredibly cathartic it can be to tell your story. And my hope is that by sharing my story I might help others as well."

As they got to know each other, Andi, in her uniquely canine way, offered emotional support—a fundamental human need as important to our mental health as food and water are to our physical survival, according to Tsai. And her support provided the boost Jessi needed not just to bounce back but to bounce *forward*. "Social support is essential to post-traumatic growth, because it buffers stress, promotes a feeling of safety, and helps people be more flexible and see their situation from a different perspective," Tsai told us. He has seen pet-inspired transformations in his studies of post-traumatic growth among veterans. "Trauma-support providers don't typically consider pets as possible aids to recovery, but they should. For some people, the companionship of animals can be integral to healing and may even lead to post-traumatic growth."

In the psychological science realm, the idea that pets can play an active role in a human's social support system is new and not widely acknowledged. But preliminary research confirms the idea that interspecies emotional support is more common than we think. When Australian researchers had 1,161 pet-owning university students complete a questionnaire designed to assess their relationships with their animal companions, they found that the students not only perceived their pets as sources of social support but that the comfort their pets provided was analogous to the nurturing they received from romantic partners, family, and friends. In their wordless way, pets helped their people feel seen, understood, and loved.

That may sound obvious to those of us who chat with our cats and confide in our dogs. But from a scientific perspective it's fairly revolutionary. Social support is indispensable for helping us not just endure life's storms but emerge from them sturdier, wiser, more compassionate, or imbued with a greater understanding of who we are and what we want to contribute to the world. Those vital connections are among the most important contributors to human health, including helping us cope with trauma—and sometimes even finding ways to *thrive*.

Animals Freed Mary From Her Painful Past

On New Year's Eve in 2002, Mary Kniskern was driving five friends from one party to the next when she lost control of her car. It was 8:45 at night, and she'd already been partying for hours. She still doesn't remember exactly how the accident happened, but she was told the vehicle flipped and rolled a hundred feet. Three passengers died. Two were her dear friends. "The word 'devastated' doesn't begin to describe how I felt," she says. "I've spent the past fifteen years of my life trying to find ways to live with the regret, guilt, sorrow, shame, and grief. There's no getting over it. I eventually realized the only thing I can do is try to honor their memory by living in a way that would make them proud."

It hasn't been easy. Mary started drinking when she was eight. Raised in a turbulent, unpredictable home, she smoked meth for the first time three years later. At thirteen, she started selling drugs to pay for clothes and food. By sixteen, she had a serious drug and alcohol habit and an adopted family of gang members, whom she had moved in with. "My mom was checked out and my stepdad wasn't a good man. Home for me meant chaos and pain. The gang was the only place I was shown love." At twenty-three, in an attempt to straighten up, she moved from San Diego to her mother's home in Sequim, Washington. "I still drank, but I had quit the hard drugs," she says. "For a few years I did okay. I got a car, a job." Then came that awful New Year's Eve that changed her life forever.

Because the police didn't charge her right away, Mary fled to California, but in 2004, the police caught up with her and put her in the Washington Corrections Center for Women in Gig Harbor, Washington, where she spent the next eight years. "It may sound strange, but once I was incarcerated, I decided to make the most of my time. I was off the streets. I was clean. I had an opportunity to change, and I was determined to take advantage of it," she says.

Not long after she arrived, she learned about the facility's Prison Pet Partnership program (PPP), a nonprofit that rescues homeless animals from all over the country and teaches inmates to train them to become service animals for people with disabilities; it also operates a boarding and grooming facility on the prison grounds to help inmates learn skills that might be beneficial once they're released. "You have to be in prison for a year before you're allowed into the program," says Mary. "I've always loved animals, from the time I was small. So one of the first things I did was get on the waiting list."

Her first job with the PPP was assessing dogs to see if they'd be a fit for the service dog training program, and she eventually earned a coveted service dog training position. "From day one, the program began to change the way I thought about myself," she says. "Those dogs depended on us to care for them and keep them healthy. I realized these abandoned, abused dogs were a lot like me. They weren't valued. They'd been given up on. And yet here I was, this discarded, hopeless person, turning abandoned, abused dogs into service animals that could change, maybe even save, people's lives. I felt needed and useful for the first time ever."

Upon her release in 2011, Mary landed a job, thanks to her experience with the Prison Pet Partnership program, at an upscale pet-grooming shop in Bellevue, Washington. A year later, she adopted a rescue dog of her own. She had gone to a local shelter to adopt a dog whose photo she'd seen online, but when she got there, a happy little bichon frise grabbed a toy, brought it to her, and lay down at her feet. "I realized he was the dog I was supposed to adopt," she says. Sonny, as she called him, was nine months old and had been found roaming the streets in Los Angeles. "He must have been through a lot, but from the minute I met him he was such a happy boy," she says. "He has these soulful eyes and is very, very, very cute. He warms everyone's heart. When I brought him home, I finally felt complete."

Not long after, she was riding in a friend's car when they were pulled over by the police, who found guns and drugs in the vehicle. In court, the judge told Mary she could avoid going back to prison if she moved to Sequim, the small town where she'd had the horrific accident, and committed to rehab. "I was terrified at how close I'd come to losing Sonny, so I knew I had to seize the opportunity to get sober," she says. "He gave me the will to change for good."

A family friend gave Mary a loan, and in July 2016 she opened Sonny's Spaw, a grooming salon. "I was nervous about opening a business in a community that had nothing but hate and disdain for me. But people were incredibly forgiving. They gave me a chance. Within a year, my business was thriving."

Since then, Mary has adopted a second dog, Stella, a one-year-old mutt who'd been abandoned as a puppy. "She was just five weeks old when I got her. Someone had dropped off a box of puppies with my old boss in Tacoma, so she called me and asked if I wanted one," says Mary. "Stella is smart and beautiful and the most difficult dog I've ever tried to train. She has no boundaries and no inhibitions. But working with her has been a blessing for both of us. She's taught me so much about patience and forgiveness and unconditional love. We're training each other.

"In my recovery, I've learned to believe that a power greater than myself can restore me to sanity," she adds. "I had to figure out what that meant, because I never had a sane life. For me, animals are an indispensable part of a balanced, sober life. The only way my life works is to be surrounded by animals."

Why Prison Pet Programs (and Their Participants) Are Thriving

When Sister Pauline Quinn, who had found emotional healing with a dog after a childhood of abuse and neglect, launched the Prison Pet Partnership Program in 1981, it was the first prison-based pet-training program in the country. Today there are as many as three hundred similar projects across the United States, many of which work with rescue animals. Most programs concentrate on training dogs, but a few feature cats. In 2016, for instance, Warm Springs

Correctional Center in Carson City, Nevada, piloted Inmates Nursing Kittens—a program that's just what it sounds like. Nevada Humane Society was overwhelmed with abandoned kittens, so they partnered with the prison to take the young felines in. The inmates nurtured the tiny creatures, feeding them from a bottle every two hours around the clock, helping them use a litter box, and giving them love and attention so they learned how to bond. When the kittens weighed two pounds, they were returned to Nevada Humane Society, where they were vaccinated, spayed or neutered, and put up for adoption. One inmate said in a news story that he felt the program was making him the man he was meant to be: "A lot of us are here because of a lack of love. With these kittens, we have learned to embrace love and to give it."

Keen to understand more about the benefits of these proliferating programs and find out if Mary's experience was typical, we contacted Barbara Cooke, PhD, assistant professor of criminal justice at Texas A&M University in Kingsville, Texas, who has been studying prison pet initiatives for seven years. "From the time I was young, my family rescued and fostered dogs, so when I heard about these programs not long before starting my master's degree in criminology, the idea stuck with me," she says.

Since then, Cooke has traveled around the country interviewing inmates and prison staff who work with dog-training programs. She also has done the most comprehensive review to date of studies looking at these programs. Together, she says, her research paints a hopeful picture of the potential for changing the direction of lost people's lives. "In general, inmates love these programs, and they cite a variety of benefits. On the most basic level, working with dogs gives them something to love and hug. You're not allowed to touch anyone in prison, and prisoners often learn not to show emotion. With the animals, they're allowed to let down their guard, and some people find that profoundly meaningful. And we know from research that hugging and petting an animal affects you on a cellular level, because it triggers your brain to release all these calming chemicals, like oxytocin and serotonin. Imagine being able to show love to an animal when you've been forced to tamp down your emotions for years. It allows inmates to open up and connect with their humanity again."

For some prisoners, like Mary, participating in the program leads to true post-traumatic growth—growth that allows them to commit to a healthier life once they're released. "A number of studies of individual programs show that recidivism is reduced among inmates who participate in these programs, and recently more comprehensive research is starting to find the same thing," says Cooke. "At this point, it appears the programs significantly reduce participants' risk of reoffending and may give them transferable skills that make them more employable when they leave prison. If that holds up to further scrutiny, it shows that these programs have the power to affect inmates on a deep, lasting level."

In a sense, the animals experience post-traumatic growth as well. They receive a second chance, during which they often become vital to the lives of the people with whom they're placed. "These programs are really a win-win-win. They help the prisoners, the animals, and the people who adopt them, whether it's someone who is disabled, a vet with PTSD, a child with autism, or an ordinary person who just wants to enjoy the love of a well-trained pet," Cooke says. "I adopted my dog, Pinto, from one of the programs. His name is a Texas slang term for people who've spent time in prison. He's a rat terrier mix, and he's one of the most well-trained dogs I've ever had. I adore him—and he got a new life thanks to the prison program."

When Grief Leads to Post-Traumatic Growth

Through my grief over losing Wilbur—which forced me to face the buried sorrow about my father's death—I experienced my own post-traumatic growth, an outcome that's not uncommon but also doesn't occur for everyone, according to Cori Bussolari, who has studied post-traumatic growth after pet loss. "The death of a loved one unsettles your core beliefs about how the world is supposed to work—and research has consistently shown that the emotional pain and social upheaval following the loss of a pet can be equal to or greater than the loss of valued people," she says. "It's that disruption of core beliefs, that feeling that your life has been turned on its head and that nothing will ever be the same, that can ultimately lead to growth."

About half of the 3,804 participants Bussolari and her team initially contacted said they'd experienced growth following the loss of a pet. Respondents said they grew in a variety of ways, from feeling more compassion for and closer to friends, family, and surviving pets, to discovering that they're stronger than they thought they were, to shifting their priorities and developing a greater appreciation for life—including living in the present the way their animal did. "The themes that emerged were remarkably similar to growth following human loss," says Bussolari.

Animals not only help us get *through* the grieving process, but due to their shorter life span, they also give us an opportunity to *practice* grieving, and to learn to let go and reconnect. In my job I see so many people who say they love their current cat or dog so much they'll never be able to get another. I might have said the same myself at one point, but enduring and working through the hurt of the loss of both Wilbur and my father taught me a lesson: There will always be a piece of my heart that belongs only to each of them. And the cats and dogs I've adopted since Wilbur passed haven't replaced him. Rather, they've expanded my heart, allowing me to become a fuller, richer, more complete human being, with a greater capacity for love.

Wilbur's death helped me understand that loneliness and isolation are barriers to experiencing the full range of what life has to offer. Animals can (and, in my opinion, should) be a pillar of your support system, but, ideally, they help you build bridges to other people whom you can rely on as well. Until then, I had defined self-sufficiency as *having* to do it alone, with my animals for support. Through my grief, I came to realize it meant being *capable* of doing it alone—and reaching out to friends and loved ones for help when I needed it. Standing on my own two feet, while remaining open and vulnerable with friends, family, and colleagues—for me, *that's* where joy lives.

After moving back to Los Altos and subsequently leaving Intuit, I took inspiration from my gregarious childhood cat, Chester, and consciously opened my heart. That's when I met Mike, a wonderful man with a soft spot for German shepherds, and fell in love. While helping me network, he introduced me to Humane Society Silicon Valley's board chair at the time, setting me on the road that led to my career today.

Through the painful experience of losing Wilbur, I learned that the courage we gain from going through the bonding cycle with animals can build our capacity to endure the same thing with the people we love and lose. It helps us enlarge and strengthen our hearts so we're ultimately able to experience love again.

Though the circumstances of Mary's situation—her incarceration and subsequent second act—were dramatically different from mine, the outcomes were surprisingly similar. In my mind, that's one of the most moving aspects of rescue animals: Their therapeutic benefits are available to everyone, regardless of background or life circumstances. Our innate connection to living creatures flows from a place that's deeply embedded in our common humanity, so the same magic has the ability to grace us all.

Jessi Burns has her own beautiful version of the narrative. After adopting Andi, she didn't just re-engage with life, she found ways to turn her tragedy into something meaningful by sharing some of what she learned with others—not only in her support groups but in the wider world as well. For instance, sharing her story with Mutual Rescue wasn't easy. It forced her to relive the most painful experience of her life. "But I chose to talk about my experience, because I wanted to open up the conversation about suicide," she says. "People turn to suicide partly because they feel so alone. I want to do my part to change that." Likewise, when she saw a listing for a job opening at an animal shelter, she saw an opportunity to help people experience the same type of growth, change, and renewal she did when she adopted Andi. "Andi was my savior," says Jessi. "She taught me to take life one day at a time and helped me stop dwelling on the past and worrying about the future. She truly saved my life—and helped me find a new one. I realized that even after terrible tragedies, beautiful things can take root and grow."

SECTION II

BODY

5

Vitalizing Physical Health

The Effect of Wags and Whiskers on Physiology

It was a sunny March day in 2015 when Matt Earnest made the seven-hour drive from his home in San Francisco to visit a friend who had just bought a new house near Los Angeles. "When I arrived, I heard a dog barking behind the house, so I walked outside, and there, in this big, dirt backyard, was a beautiful, friendly six-year-old golden retriever," recalls Matt. The dog's name was Samson. He belonged to Matt's friend's brother, who was living in a condo where he couldn't have the dog—a situation that was supposed to be temporary. "My buddy told me that as soon as his brother found a new house, he'd take Samson again," recalls Matt, now thirty-five. "In the meantime, Samson was usually outside, because my friend and his girlfriend had cats. If he was inside, he was in a crate. I felt bad for the poor guy, so I spent most of my visit out back playing fetch with him. Samson didn't have the life he deserved, and he seemed a little sad. When I left, he and I both cried. I promised him I'd be back."

Matt could relate to the dog's unhappiness. At the time, he was just pulling out of a major depression of his own, a sudden, scary downward spiral brought on partly by a career crisis. Like Samson, Matt felt hemmed in by circumstance. In his early thirties, with no college degree, and interesting but disparate job skills, he was still trying to figure out what he wanted to do with his life—and he was worried that his options were limited. "In my twenties, I'd spent a few years organizing raves and music festivals. I'd worked at Disney, and I'd worked at Lyft as director of special events and community logistics. But I left in January to attend a tech school in hopes of finding a new career path. When I realized it wasn't right for me, I completely fell apart and felt like giving up on everything, including life," he says. "By the time I met Samson I was no longer danger-ously depressed, but I was unhealthy. I weighed two hundred sixty pounds and was eating and drinking and partying too much in an attempt to make myself feel better."

Matt made good on his parting promise to Samson. Every month, he got in his car and hit the road for the long drive to Los Angeles. With each visit, their bond grew. When Matt arrived in July, he found the seventy-pound dog outside by himself in the 100-degree weather. "He had plenty of water, but I was concerned, and it broke my heart to see him alone," he says. "By the end of that visit, I'd made a decision: I put Samson in my car and told my buddy I was going to take him home to live with me until his brother figured out his housing situation."

Having Samson around on a daily basis made Matt feel more grounded, and, even though he wasn't sure he was going to be able to keep the dog, he committed to training him. "Samson was so smart and so grateful to me for giving him a home that before long, I could walk him without a leash and he'd stay by my side," he says. "We built this crazy connection, and I could see how good he was for me emotionally. Being with Samson took me out of the haunted places in my head and helped me start feeling more positive."

By January 2016, it was clear that Samson's owner wouldn't be asking for him back. He was officially Matt's dog. Feeling more stable emotionally, Matt landed a job at a tech company, and on his lunch hour he started extending his walks with his energetic dog from short strolls to two-mile loops. Two miles quickly turned into five, then into seven or eight. "Every time we increased our distance, I felt more confident about my ability to set and attain goals—and Samson loved our outings. He was up for anything. He could just go and go and go," says Matt. "The cool and surprising thing I discovered was that all that exercise was good for my brain. I could feel my negative thoughts start to change. Instead of telling myself life was hopeless, I started seeing possibilities again. Before my depression, I had been an energetic, enthusiastic guy. Samson reminded me what that looks like. He was healing me, one walk at a time."

One Sunday morning in mid-February, Matt woke up with a killer hangover. "I took Samson out and we just started walking. We ended up doing this massive sixteen-mile loop around the city, so I had plenty of time to think, and I began trying to figure out what was holding me back from fulfilling my career and life potential. One of the major factors, I realized, was my health. My weight, my partying, my poor eating habits had all gotten out of control. I'd been living on pizza, burritos, beer, and carbs, carbs, carbs. By the time we got home, my hangover was gone, and in its place was a new resolution to get healthy."

Matt began increasing his walking distance and added running to the mix. By the summer of 2016, he and Samson were logging fifty to sixty miles a week—and he had lost thirty pounds. "My mood was better than ever, and the more I exercised, the less I craved pizza and crappy food," he says. "I started snacking on veggies and hummus and eating things like kale salad, something I never would have done before. I was feeding Samson super healthy food, too. We were both getting stronger and healthier."

That summer, Matt landed an exciting new job at General Motors—a step that made him feel like his life was back on track. "Samson is doing great, too. I had him certified as a psychiatric service dog. If I start getting upset or angry, he barks at me and reminds me to calm down. We've both grown and changed, and our relationship is incredibly tight. We trust each other and take care of each other and love each other. And a big part of that mutual care is a commitment to better health. Neither of us could have done it alone. Together, we're able to stay on track."

The New Rx for Heart Health: Adopt a Pet

With the success of *Eric & Peety*, our first Mutual Rescue film, about an obese man who lost weight after adopting a shelter dog (see page 84), we were curious if other people had experienced similar benefits and posted the question on Facebook. That's when we received Matt's before and after photos and heard about his inspiring metamorphosis—more proof that pets can be a powerful catalyst for healthy lifestyle changes.

Even better, when we started looking at research, we found Matt's heartwarming anecdote is actually grounded in science. In fact, research on the therapeutic role pets can play in cardiovascular health is so promising that, in 2013, the American Heart Association (AHA) issued a scientific statement, in which it reviewed all the studies to date and concluded that pet ownership, particularly dog ownership, is "probably associated" with a decreased risk of cardiovascular disease.

"Probably associated" may not sound like a ringing endorsement, but medical organizations are conservative in their approach and opinions. Doctors don't go in for superlatives, and science doesn't always yield definitive answers. For instance, a 2017 AHA review of the effect of meditation, a widely endorsed stress reliever on cardiovascular risk reduction, found there was a "possible benefit." In truth, the fact that the AHA looked at the research on animals and heart health at all is unusual—and the group's cautiously positive take-away borders on stunning. If the science on pets' effect on heart health is solid enough to persuade one of the most powerful nonprofit health advocacy groups in the country, that should get our attention. What's more, endorsements from the AHA are influential. As the nation's largest cardiovascular health organization, its views hold sway with doctors and can guide their treatment recommendations. And when general practitioners and internists become enthusiastic about an approach, it can affect the well-being of untold numbers of people who are suffering from poor health and searching for solutions.

A year after the AHA endorsement, an online panel survey of 1,000 family doctors and general practitioners from around the country found evidence that physicians *are* getting on board. A full 60 percent of doctors surveyed said they have recommended pet adoption to patients to improve their overall health as well as for a specific purpose, like alleviating depression, encouraging physical activity, and reducing stress. In addition, 75 percent said they had seen one or more of their patients' health improve after adopting a pet, 87 percent reported that they'd seen an uptick in patients' mood or outlook—and an impressive 97 percent said they believe there are health benefits of owning a pet.

"We all know that eating our veggies and getting regular exercise are important for our health. Now the majority of physicians say pets should be on that list," says Steven Feldman, executive director of the Human Animal Bond Research Institute (HABRI), the organization that commissioned the survey. We contacted Feldman because, as the head of HABRI, a nonprofit created in 2010 to fund and disseminate research on the therapeutic effect of pets, he has his finger on the pulse of human-animal science as a whole. While HABRI obviously has a pro-animal agenda (it was founded by the American Pet Products Association, Zoetis, and Petco), part of its mission is to get high-quality, unbiased research into the public sphere. "The only way for the field to move forward and to learn the truth about the benefits of animals is with impartial, gold-standard research. At this point, not all studies on the human-animal bond meet that bar. But if we want to convince people that pets are as helpful as we believe they are, we need to show it with objective science," Feldman says. "For example, the outcome of studies on heart health shows a correlation between pets and improved cardiovascular health, including lower blood pressure and reduced stress. They support the idea that having animals in our lives is protective. That's a mind-set shift. We've gone from believing that pets are nice to have around to understanding that they actually can play an important role in our health and wellness."

New solutions to address the lifestyle habits and other factors that contribute to heart disease, like lack of exercise, poor diet, high blood pressure, and the tragic epidemic of obesity, couldn't be more needed. More than 70 percent of adults in the United States are overweight or obese, according to the Centers for Disease Control, and just 51 percent meet the recommended 150 minutes of moderate aerobic activity per week.

Being overweight can lead to chronic low-grade, systemic inflammation, a key risk factor for cardiovascular disease (CVD), an illness that exacts a terrible price. CVD is the underlying cause of about 800,000 deaths in the United States every year, making it the number one killer, claiming more lives than cancer and chronic respiratory disease combined. On average, one person every forty seconds succumbs to the illness—and 92 million adults are currently living with some form of the disease. If adopting a pet could ease even a small part of the problem, it would be a tremendous boon for society. And there's growing consensus that it can.

The first study to find a link between companion animals and heart health was published in 1980, when researchers at the University of Pennsylvania documented an association between pet ownership and a significant decrease in mortality in the year following a heart attack or an episode of chest pain. Of the thirty-nine patients in the study who didn't own a pet, eleven died a year after the event. Of the fifty-three who did have an animal companion, all but three were still alive a year later. The analysis was small, but it hinted at a profoundly meaningful association between owning a pet and protecting your heart—an association that has, in a number of studies since, been borne out.

Research papers have found that people who have pets may have healthier cholesterol levels, lower blood pressure, and a less extreme reaction to stress than those who don't—all of which can help keep your cardiovascular system trouble-free. Those benefits can translate into better health—and can even add years to your life. One study found that cat owners have a 30 percent lower risk of heart attack compared to non–cat owners, probably because they help reduce stress and blood pressure. Another that looked at nearly 4,000 people age fifty and older found that women who owned a cat had a significantly lower risk of dying of a cardiovascular-related event, particularly a stroke, than non–cat owners.

Meanwhile, Swedish investigators have conducted by far the largest exploration of the association between dog ownership and human health to date. They combed through twelve years of health data from 3.4 million people ages forty to eighty, 13 percent of whom owned a dog, and found that dog owners who lived alone were, on average, 33 percent less likely to die of any cause and 11 percent less likely to die of a heart attack than those without a dog. Dog owners who lived with others had an 11 percent lower risk of dying of any cause and a 15 percent lower risk of succumbing to cardiovascular disease—a remarkable finding that's encouraging for all of us who share a home with an exuberant, drooling beast or two.

Heart disease is complex. There's no single solution that will alleviate this national health crisis or work for everyone. But while statins and blood pressure medications chip away at discrete aspects of the problem, more people—and more doctors—are discovering what Matt learned: that a pet can change your *attitude* toward your health, inspire you to revamp your habits, and often bolster your motivation and commitment to the lifestyle changes that are essential in order to fully regain your health.

The Story That Launched Mutual Rescue—and Captured the World's Heart

The first time I came to truly appreciate the impact homeless animals can have on seriously ill people, altering the lives of those who are dangerously obese and who've all but given up hope of ever regaining their health, was when I heard about Eric O'Grey. Several years before we started Mutual Rescue, we received an astonishing email from Eric, who had adopted a dog from Humane Society Silicon Valley the year before.

When he first walked into the shelter, Eric weighed 340 pounds, had dangerously high cholesterol and type 2 diabetes, and was socially withdrawn. His doctor had warned him that if he didn't revamp his lifestyle, he'd be dead within five years. Eric ignored him. After all, he'd tried and failed on every diet out there. What could possibly help? Then, while traveling for business, Eric's plane had to delay its departure so flight attendants could find him a seat belt extension. The irate passenger next to him said, "I'm going to miss my flight because you're too fat." Something about that moment broke through Eric's inertia and prompted him to call a new physician, Preeti Kulkarni, ND, a naturopathic doctor, for help. Her first piece of advice: Adopt a shelter dog to help you get out and exercise. "I ask patients on their intake form whether they have a pet, and if they don't, I often suggest they adopt one—whether it's to bolster their commitment to regular physical activity or for companionship or stress relief," says Dr. Kulkarni. "Not a single patient who has acted on that recommendation has regretted it. I firmly believe that pets can play an important role in health and wellness."

As it happened, we had the perfect match for Eric. Peety, a border collie mix, had been struggling, too, before coming into the shelter. He had itchy skin from untreated dermatitis and was also overweight. Together, he and Eric began to exercise. Eventually, Eric lost 150 pounds and reversed all his health problems, including his diabetes, while Peety shed twenty-five pounds. Not only that, he and Peety, he told us, had formed a devoted bond. "I'd never experienced anything like it with another living soul, human or animal," he said. "That relationship made me a different person. I became more empathetic and more in tune with the suffering of others."

When we decided to make short films for Mutual Rescue, his

journey with Peety was the first one we created. The world fell in love with *Eric & Peety*. Since the film's release in February 2016, it has been viewed more than 100 million times. But the thing I find so heartwarming about Eric's remarkable path from life-threatening obesity to paragon of fitness is that it can be traced back to a single tender moment: When a forlorn and ailing human saw shades of himself in a chubby, eager-to-please, middle-aged dog and decided to give him a home.

Why Pets Have the Power to Transform Human Health

Science is still exploring the hows and whys of pets' effects on heart health, but it's likely that several factors intermingle synergistically to create a web of protective benefits. For one thing, cats and dogs can calm us down and smooth the jagged edges of stress, minimizing the damaging toll the stress hormone, cortisol, has on our hearts (it is known for increasing blood pressure and cholesterol as well as causing weight gain) and enlarging our ability to experience joy.

During my lonely time in Santa Rosa, I could actually feel my heart rate drop and my body begin to relax as I petted Wilbur and Wiley—signs that real physiological changes were taking place beneath my skin. As I stroked their soft fur, the thrum of their purrs resonating beneath my fingers, my heart rhythm was likely synchronizing with theirs into a relaxing pattern. Two research groups in the past decade, one in the United States and the other in Australia, have shown that animals' and humans' hearts start beating in synchrony when they spend time together—a phenomenon known as heart coherence—providing preliminary evidence that rescue pets don't just change our behavior; their life-affirming influence burrows deep into our body's biorhythms, giving both animals and humans a respite from worry and providing physical renewal and relief.

By conferring a greater sense of ease and reducing cortisol, pets may also enhance our ability to make healthy food choices. Because cortisol is the hormone underlying our body's fight-or-flight mode, it's designed to ensure we have plenty of fuel on board to do battle or flee. It stealthily, subconsciously undermines our resolve to eat healthfully. It intensifies appetite, recent research shows, as well as the urge to eat, even if you don't feel hungry. As distressing, it increases cravings for foods that are high in saturated fat and sugar, the very things most of us are trying to avoid.

A second path by which pets seem to improve our heart health is by encouraging exercise—and in this realm, dogs shine. They crave physical activity. Undeterred by inclement weather, bad moods, work deadlines, or the soporific lure of the sofa, they're the species most likely to nudge us out of the house—often by placing their damp muzzles in our laps and staring up at us with pleading eyes or prancing around in front of the door, leash in mouth.

By capitulating to our canines' blatant pleas for outdoor time (which many dog owners seem to do, seeing as they're 55 percent more likely than non–dog owners to get the recommended amount of daily exercise) we get far more than we give, because movement, quite simply, is medicine. Physical activity affects nearly every biological factor that leads to heart disease. It helps with weight control, strengthens the heart, improves circulation, and reduces blood pressure, blood sugar, and triglycerides, or fat in your blood. As Rebecca Johnson, PhD, director of the Human–Animal Interaction Research Center at the University of Missouri College of Veterinary Medicine, told us: "Exercise is good for both ends of the leash."

Johnson, who has studied animals' effects on human health for twenty-five years, knows as much as anyone on the topic. Her research has found, for instance, that walking dogs can help people commit to exercise and lose weight. In one experiment, she and a colleague recruited twenty-six public housing residents, all of whom were sedentary and overweight, to walk dogs for twenty minutes five days a week. In a finding that gives new meaning to the word "shedding," participants who stuck with the dog-walking program for twenty-six weeks lost an average of five pounds, while those who continued for fifty weeks lost an average of more than fourteen pounds.

"Without even discussing nutrition, we helped participants lose a healthy amount of weight and improve their physical functioning. It was gratifying to see how much their fitness improved. Some of the participants couldn't even walk fifty feet at the beginning of the study, and by the time they'd been doing it nine months they were walking one hour five days a week," she says. "Part of the reason the intervention was effective is that participants felt committed to the dogs—the same reason many people who have dogs of their own are more likely to exercise."

Walking isn't just good for the body, it's a balm for the brain, triggering the release of healthy chemicals that can help you feel more optimistic, more hopeful, more self-assured, less stressed. Those benefits, associated with movement itself, are augmented by other factors unique to dog walking. "Taking a stroll with your dog gets you outside, which can lower stress and bolster mood, and gives you the opportunity to interact with neighbors and other people you come across along the way—and social contact is good for your mood and health, too," says Johnson. The mood elevation that exercise provides may be another reason why walking with their dogs— a single, simple lifestyle change—galvanized both Matt and Eric to start taking better care of themselves in other ways, cleaning up their diets and minimizing alcohol.

Given the multiplicity of benefits, it's somewhat surprising that up to 40 percent of dog owners rarely walk their pets—a missed opportunity for humans and canines alike, given the pleasures and perks of the shared experience. Over the past few years, Carri Westgarth, PhD, a research fellow in human–animal interaction at the University of Liverpool in England, has focused her research on identifying the factors that prevent people from indulging in this low-intensity yet profoundly healthy ritual.

Convenience is a factor, of course, as is weather. No surprise there. What was more unexpected: Many dog owners, in a roundabout way, blamed their canines. "If we think our dogs don't enjoy walking, we don't enjoy it, either—and can easily make excuses not to bother," says Westgarth. As a result, smaller dogs and older, heavier canines, she found, are less likely to get out for a stroll, because people tell themselves they don't like or need to be walked. "But it's not true that small dogs don't need walks," insists Westgarth, whose own Chihuahua-pug mix has gamely accompanied her to the top of the 3,500-foot peak of Mount Snowdon in Wales. "And, while you might need to take shorter, slower walks with older or overweight dogs, you can still take them. People should ask themselves: Is it really my dog who's too tired to go for a walk or is it me?"

Committed dog walkers, on the other hand, often feel a sense of duty to their dogs' well-being. "The powerful two-way interaction we have with our dogs, and the reciprocal and unconditional nature of the love we get from them, engenders a sense of responsibility for many dog owners," says Westgarth.

And sometimes the sheer pleasure of sharing an excursion with an ecstatic hound is enough to get people out the door. There's no joy like seeing your dog spin in exuberant circles—and their glee is evidently contagious. "Our studies have shown that the number one reason people walk their dogs is because it makes them—the *humans*—happy," explains Westgarth, who is currently investigating how much extra physical activity dog owners get thanks to their canines. (Hint: "The payoff looks to be huge," she says.) "In this age of information and work overload, we have our dogs to thank for getting us outside, letting us share their abundant joy and providing a sense of balance and well-being."

Just as spending time with a friend deepens your relationship, sharing lighthearted outings with your dog helps strengthen your bond—and that lovely feeling of closeness with your canine, the reassuring sense that he or she loves you unreservedly (a feeling that we receive from cats as well), can *also* help safeguard your heart. Researchers have discovered receptors for oxytocin, the calming hormone of love and bonding, in all four chambers of the heart as well as the blood vessels surrounding this vital organ. When you interact with your treasured pet, molecules of oxytocin click into the receptors embedded deep in your chest and work their magic, slowing your heart rate, relaxing your blood vessels, and lowering your blood pressure—all of which help protect the pulsing structure that keeps you alive.

Think about that the next time you're deciding whether you have the time or energy to stroll around the block or along a trail with your dog. Those sniffing, wagging, meandering forays are more than exercise. In ways both tangible and ineffable, they lift your heart itself.

No Dog? No Problem! You Can Walk a Shelter Dog

At the University of Missouri, Johnson has done a number of studies, but there is one that brings me particular joy: a seven-year study called Walk a Hound, Lose a Pound. For the study, they enrolled community residents in Columbia, Missouri, to walk a shelter dog at Central Missouri Humane Society every Saturday for a month. That's it. Four walks and each participant was done. "We tracked people afterward and found that after just four Saturdays of dog walking, people started parking their cars farther from their destination or taking the stairs more often or walking around the block with their partners after dinner. It helped them do more exercise overall. In behavior change, there's a contemplation stage, where you're thinking about doing something, and there's the action phase, where you follow through on your plans. Walking a shelter dog once a week was enough to move a number of our participants from contemplation to action."

At Humane Society Silicon Valley, we launched a similar program in 2016 to give our larger dogs a break from the confines of the shelter and offer people who don't own a dog the opportunity to spend quality time with one. Called Doggy Day Out, it encourages people from the community to take a rescue dog on an outing to the beach, the local hiking trails, or home for a hangout. (There are many shelters across the country doing these kinds of programs. Please visit MutualRescue.org/Doggy-Day-Out to find a program at a local shelter in your area.)

Susannah Greenwood, forty-three, of San Jose, California, who has two rescue cats but grew up with a dog, started participating in Doggy Day Out not long after the program started—and has been doing it almost every week ever since. "When I took my first shelter dog out, I'd just been let go from a job and my soulmate cat had recently passed away, so I was hurting across the spectrum, from personally to professionally," she says. "I saw a post about Doggy Day Out on Facebook and thought it would give me a nice break from sitting at home and stressing about my résumé."

On her first visit, Susannah was paired with a gorgeous, energetic pit bull named Layla. "I took her on a local trail that was wet and muddy from the rain, and she was so happy she just wanted to run," Susannah recalls. "I was out of shape and couldn't keep up with her, so I ended up taking her to my backyard. As I was hosing her off, she started playing and splashing around in the water. She looked so adorable I pulled out my phone and filmed her. The shelter posted the video on its Facebook page, and Layla was adopted the next day. I was hooked."

Susannah, who now works in marketing for an arts organization, says, "Being with a shelter dog boosts my mood and motivates me to push myself physically—and I feel good about doing it, because it's clearly so fun for the dogs," she says. When she started hiking with the dogs, she struggled to do a mile and a half. Now she routinely hikes four or five miles without a problem. "It feels great to sweat. It clears my mind. It helps me sleep. It brings me real joy. Exercise is cleansing, emotionally and physically," she says. "When I first signed up for the Doggy Day Out program I did it because I wanted to give a gift to the dogs. I quickly realized I was the one who was reaping the real benefits. It's a win-win every time."

Matt and Eric would undoubtedly agree. Their experiences point to a deeper insight about animals and heart health: The answer to our health and weight problems may lie not in external fixes, like diets and punishing exercise routines, but in feeling good about ourselves. "I had the opportunity to see Eric transform from a man who could barely look me in the eye to an outgoing, engaged, active, confident human being," says Dr. Kulkarni. Having a close relationship with a rescue pet helps you feel not just loved, but *lovable*.

An adoring cat or dog isn't guaranteed to shore up shaky self-esteem and make you want to take better care of your health. But there are millions of us around the world who can vouch for the fact it can. "Everything started coming together for me after I adopted Samson," says Matt. "My mood improved, I started exercising and eating better, and I'm now two hundred five pounds, a healthy weight for my six-foot-one frame. I even got sober. People struggle for years to make these kinds of changes—and it took effort for me, too. But having Samson made the effort seem worth it."

Eric's reflections are similar. Before meeting Peety, not even the fear of dying was enough to motivate him to turn his health around, but an abandoned dog gave him something no diet book or nutritionist could. As Eric explains it, "Peety taught me the meaning of friendship and how to love myself. He helped me believe in myself again. Peety thought I was the greatest—so I decided to become the person he thought I was."

6

Embracing Joy

Animals' Playful Companionship Transforms Loneliness

For most of her life, Judy Torigoe, a seventy-two-year-old piano teacher in Cottonwood, Arizona, lived alone—happily. She was proud of her independence, loved her career, and never had the sense that anything was missing from her life. Then in 2006, her mom died, and she inherited Josh, her mother's nine-year-old cockapoo. "It took us a few months to establish our relationship, because he was totally spoiled. But once we did, we bonded—*strongly*. I had no idea I could get that close to a dog," she says.

Three years later, when Josh died, her grief shook her so deeply it scared her. "I dreamed about Josh and woke up in the middle of the night calling his name," she says. "I could hardly eat or sleep. I actually stood in the middle of the living room one day and screamed, 'I want my baby back!' I was in such despair I didn't know what to do. Nothing relieved it. People suggested getting another dog. I was horrified. I thought of it as trying to replace Josh. When he died, it was like the best part of me was gone. I felt like life would never be the same again."

She swore she'd never get another animal. The pain of the loss was simply too great. Her resolve lasted just three weeks.

"Without Josh, I saw what loneliness felt like—and it was awful," she says. "I felt so alone it frightened me. For the first time in life, my choice to remain single and childless began to haunt me. My family is small. I don't even have cousins. Josh had given me a sense of companionship I never knew I was missing. Without him, I needed something—*someone*—to fill the hole he left in my life."

She began searching for another small dog at the shelters in her area, but couldn't find one that was right for her, so in desperation she cast a wider net, then wider still. Finally, she located several poodle mixes at Animal Rescue League of El Paso in Texas. The shelter was 550 miles away from her home at the time in Sedona, Arizona. She didn't care. She got in her car and drove south the next day.

When she got to the shelter, she spotted a small white poodle mix, with long, floppy ears and a wise, kind face. The sweet-looking one-year-old girl had been spayed the day before, so she was subdued, but Judy remembered this dog from the photos she'd seen on the website. The dog's bio, which Judy had printed out while she was researching potential pets, said: "I get along with other dogs, like to play, like to be petted and want to be loved forever. Adopt me today and find a friend for life." Next to the bio were three photos of the little white dog smiling from ear to ear. Under the photos, Judy had scrawled a two-word note to herself: *Definite possibility.*

Judy asked if she could take the grinning dog out of her crate. Once she did, the pup went from possibility to sure thing. "There was something about her calm demeanor and the way she always found the softest spot to lie down that made me think we'd get along well," Judy says. She signed the adoption papers and named the fluffy white pup Yuki, the Japanese word, when used as a name, for happiness.

Both she and Yuki were anxious during the long drive back to Arizona. When they finally made it home, the first thing Yuki did when Judy set her loose in the house was poop. *Three* times. "I had to laugh," says Judy. "I knew the trip had been as stressful for her as it had for me. It was a slightly rocky start, but I took her out for our first walk not long after and experienced pure joy. Yuki was eager to immerse herself in all the new smells on our street. Watching her get to know her new home over the next days and weeks was so gratifying. I still loved Josh as much as ever, but being with Yuki made me miss him less."

As they got to know each other better, Judy realized her new companion must have been abused as a puppy. "To this day, Yuki cringes every time I reach down to put her halter on, and she recoils if she thinks I'm angry with her. My heart aches to think of what her life must have been like before we were together."

In the safety of Judy's care, however, Yuki blossomed. "She's such a happy little creature. When she wants attention, she'll come and look up at me and wag her little tail furiously, with that same adorable grin on her face. It's simply irresistible."

Having Yuki in her home brought Judy back to life again, too. "After I lost Josh, I felt terribly lonely, like I only had half a life. The house was silent. I no longer had to walk or feed the dog. You don't realize how much those activities shape your life until they're gone. Once I adopted Yuki I had someone to care for again," says Judy. "She's the reason I get out of bed. I know she's waiting for me and needs me—and I love that feeling. There's something deeply satisfying about being needed. Her companionship has been a blessing. She never complains. She's never demanding. She can read my facial expressions and body language. We're in sync. She's like the child I never had. Together, we're a family."

Our Biological Need for Connection

We humans are a social lot. Nearly everything, from despair to delight, is bettered when we share it. When we face challenges, we instinctively turn to trusted confidants for help. When we're frightened or worried, we huddle together, finding shelter in the presence of others. Even when we're happy, we yearn to celebrate our elation with friends and family. We laugh harder and immerse more fully in the joy of play when we have an ally by our side.

Our earliest ancestors evolved to survive in tribes. Without adequate weapons, their only real protection from predators was one another. Those who were ostracized often perished. At some point, millennia ago, our brains developed biological systems designed to keep us safely embedded in families and clans. (Dogs, too, share our pack mentality—which may be one reason our two species get along so famously.) To this day, we humans are wired to seek out and maintain bonds.

The isolated among us are no longer at risk of being devoured by a saber-toothed tiger, but they might as well be. Chronic loneliness can be almost as deadly. In 2016, researchers from the United Kingdom pooled data from twenty-three studies and found that social isolation or feelings of loneliness increased the risk of having a heart attack or stroke by about 30 percent, making loneliness as perilous as smoking. In a separate meta-analysis of three million people, loneliness increased the odds of early death by 26 percent. Its health effects can be so serious that, in 2018, the United Kingdom actually appointed a minister of loneliness in response to research showing that more than 9 million people in the country often or always feel lonesome.

Feeling isolated is dangerous, because it trips an ancient biological warning signal in our brains—the same one that's triggered by hunger or thirst or pain—generating a cascade of physiological reactions designed to motivate us to go out and make friends. John Cacioppo, PhD, director of the Center for Cognitive and Social Neuroscience at the University of Chicago, who conducted a number of studies on loneliness, pointed out that from that perspective, loneliness is a symptom of a lack of social connection, just like thirst is a symptom of not having enough to drink. Heed the warning and connect with others, and the system turns off, just like hunger goes away when you eat. Ignore its message, as the chronically isolated do, and the biological consequences can ravage the body and mind.

There's a reason solitary confinement has long been used as a form of punishment. Loneliness is associated with depression, diminished cognitive control, psychosis, and suicide. It interferes with our immune system's ability to fight infection, accelerates cognitive decline, disrupts sleep, causes our bodies to age more quickly, and triggers a surge of stress hormones and inflammation, putting us at increased risk of heart disease, diabetes, and arthritis.

If we still lived in a society in which social isolation was rare—where families had homes within blocks of one another, friends stopped by every day to visit, and neighbors knew and touched base with each other regularly—loneliness wouldn't be a public health threat. But as many as 42.6 million American adults over age forty-five are estimated to be suffering from chronic loneliness, according to a study by the American Association of Retired Persons. Surprisingly, they found rates were more than 50 percent higher in younger age groups than older; 43 percent of respondents in their forties said they were lonely, compared to just 25 percent of those seventy and older. Other studies have found that children, teens, and twenty- and thirty-somethings are increasingly affected as well, as technology and social media make us all more apt to interact with our screens than with one another. As Britain's prime minister, Theresa May, said in explaining why she felt it important to address the problem, loneliness is the "sad reality of modern life."

But Judy's story reveals that there's reason for hope. In shelters across the country, millions of eager but forgotten cats and dogs are in need of companionship, too. Adopting a homeless pet might not cure the epidemic of loneliness sweeping the world, but it can provide individuals who feel socially or emotionally isolated with the sense that someone is in their corner—and has the potential to help untold numbers of lovable felines and canines find new homes.

An Imperfect Cat Can Be a Perfect Companion

Lis Phelps was twenty-four and living in Portland, Oregon, far from her family in the Midwest, when her life began to unravel. She'd quit her high-stress job at a call center, determined to return to school full-time, and not long after that, her boyfriend left her. She was broke, overwhelmed, and reeling from her breakup, which had left her without a place to live. "I'd had a happy life—and suddenly I was alone with nothing left to my name except for a handful of boxes. I was worried about how I was going to survive and still finish school."

The only bright spot in her life was her cat, Ishtar. When Lis was still living in the Midwest, her grandmother, who knew Lis loved animals, had offered to pay the fees for Lis to adopt a cat for her twentieth birthday. She went to PetSmart, which was hosting a local shelter pet expo, where one of the six available felines caught her eye. The quirky character had one green eye and one brown, her unruly fur stood out all over the place, giving her a semi-wild appearance, and even though she was thirteen months old, she was barely bigger than the kitten in the kennel next to her. "She didn't really fit the perfect cat mold, but I didn't feel like I fit the human mold, either, so I thought we should meet. I asked to hold her, and she crawled onto my shoulder and curled up against the fleece collar of my jacket," Lis recalls. "For ten minutes, I walked around with her purring in my ear, and when I tried to let someone else hold her she clung to my jacket and wouldn't let go. I said, 'Sorry, it looks like this cat has claimed me' and went to sign the adoption papers."

Ishtar turned out to be unlike any cat Lis had ever known. "She wasn't aloof or skittish at all. She was such an easygoing companion and so fun to be around—and I was able to take her everywhere," Lis says. "After I lost my job and my boyfriend, I couldn't afford rent so I was couch-surfing, and Ishtar happily moved from apartment to apartment."

Even so, Lis felt disconnected from humanity. "I had friends, but I couldn't go out at night because I didn't have any money, and I didn't have anyone I could really talk to or share my fears with," Lis recalls. "I felt like an inconvenience and a burden to my friends, and I had nowhere to call home. I spent many days locked in my room, lying in bed crying. Ishy would crawl on top of me and lick away my tears. I can still feel the sensation of her lying on my chest. I'd be thinking that there was no hope and no one I could turn to for help, but Ishy would nose my face and lick my tears and give me this look, like, 'Stop that! I'm right here.' She forced me to listen to her. Her friendship and love kept me going. She was the only thing that gave me a sense of hope."

After mulling her options, Lis chose to do something she'd long rejected: move back in with her parents in Kansas. "Ishy and I had sort of run out of couches to surf, and I really wanted a better life for her. We both needed more support and stability, and the only way we were going to get that was if *I* made some changes—and I figured the best place to start was reconnecting with old friends and family," she says.

Being home wasn't easy at first, but it felt good to see old friends, and she began to meet new ones as well. She and Ishtar moved into a tiny studio apartment a few months after being home, and by the time she'd been in Kansas a year, Lis met a man through an online community and fell in love. Then she landed a job in digital marketing. Now she owns a house, is in a stable, loving relationship, and has a fulfilling career.

"Without Ishy I'm not sure any of this would have happened," says Lis. "She was more than just a pet. She was my friend, my constant companion, my lifeline. At a time when I was lonelier than I've ever been, she was there for me. Her attachment to me, her belief in me, and her constant love and presence were the things I clung to. They were the things that helped me believe I'd be able to find a better life. It took a while to convince me. But once I finally took action to change my circumstances, my life began to improve."

In 2016, Lis suffered another heartbreak, when her beloved Ishtar was diagnosed with terminal cancer. Watching her happy-go-lucky cat lose weight and become withdrawn and lethargic was wrenching. "She'd always been so *there*, such a constant in my life and so much a part of me and who I am. When she was gone, my mind had trouble accepting it. For weeks, I'd automatically call her name, and

I still miss her every single day," says Lis. "She saw me through the lowest point of my life. She was my savior and my best friend, a tiny guardian who latched on to me and wouldn't let go. By the time she passed, I think she knew her work was done. I was finally happy. It was safe for her to move on."

The Social Support of Pets Can Actually Change Our Biology

In most ways, Lis and Judy couldn't be more different. But the sense of isolation that caused their suffering was the same, as was the remedy for their pain. A feral-looking cat and a buoyant dog made each woman, young and old, feel less lonely and alone—a story that plays out in homes across the country and is now showing up in the data of scientific studies. Over the past couple of decades, research has revealed that the camaraderie of a pet can ease loneliness in diverse groups—isolated HIV patients, older women, rural adolescents from ethnically diverse backgrounds, residents of long-term care facilities.

"It comes down to a biochemical response," explains Rebecca Johnson, director of the Research Center for Human-Animal Interaction at the University of Missouri, who conducted the walking study we talked about in Chapter 5. "We live in a high-tech, low-touch world, but, like our relationships with people, pets give us the opportunity to engage our senses—touch, sight, smell, hearing—which triggers the release of all sorts of beneficial neurochemicals that are associated with bonding and close relationships."

Stroking our animals' fur and looking into their eyes reduces the stress hormone cortisol and releases oxytocin, the bonding hormone. Taking care of an animal—feeding it, brushing it—triggers the release of prolactin, the hormone related to breast-feeding that produces a feeling of nurturing and being nurtured. Awash in these chemicals of affiliation, we feel more at ease, more connected, more in touch with something bigger than ourselves—like being enveloped in the comforting hug of a friend.

A strong connection with a companion animal can sustain you through periods when you feel unable to relate to people in your life. And enjoying the company of pets can help you stay interpersonally engaged, so when the time is right, you can again develop rapport and build fulfilling relationships with people.

Chris Blazina, PhD, a psychologist in New Mexico who studies the human–animal bond, told us the phenomenon might be particularly helpful for men. A psychologist for more than twenty years, he specializes in the emotional lives of males and explained, "Men's social circles tend to shrink when they age, and they run the risk of shutting down emotionally, which can isolate them further." But some men are more able to be open and vulnerable with animals, giving them the practice they need to remain open and engaged with people.

Chris has had that experience himself. In his late thirties, he developed Ménière's disease, an illness that causes uncontrollable bouts of vertigo and vomiting and throws off sufferers' balance and hearing, making it difficult to function—especially to communicate. The disorder struck not long after his rescue dog, Kelsey, passed away. While he was already buckling under the heaviness of his grief, the illness drove him deeper into isolation. "I basically retreated from the world," he says. "I didn't know how to deal with my grief, and when I began to get sick I was so miserable that I pushed people away. But my rescue dog, Sadie, a border collie, was a constant presence. She was my existential grounding. We'd go for a walk in the woods in the morning and again in the afternoon. And when I had an episode of vomiting, she'd sit in the bathroom with me, watching and waiting for the attack to end. It was tempting to fall into a black hole. But walking with Sadie and having her in my life helped me track my way out."

One of the things Sadie did, he says, was preserve a sense of hope that he'd be able to have meaningful attachments again with people. "Without her, I'm not sure that would have happened. I might have resigned myself to being a bachelor. By being such a loyal companion, Sadie kept that hardwired desire for connection alive. When I met my wife in my early forties, I still had the inclination, thanks to Sadie, to reach out and invite her in."

Sadie was so single-mindedly devoted to Chris, she didn't warm to his wife immediately. "So my wife had a talk with Sadie and said, 'If you let me into your circle I promise I'll never leave Chris for the rest of my life.' Sadie became closer to my wife after that, and when our son, Harris, was born, Sadie adored him."

Animals Turn Strangers into Friends

The idea that animals can facilitate your ability to form human relationships is an angle researchers have explored as well. Being with pets can help children and adults with autism build social skills, for instance—a topic we'll plumb more deeply in future chapters. And animals help link lonely people with other humans in a far more concrete and practical way as well. People who walk their dogs (or cats, as some do) have more social contact. They stop and chat with neighbors or passersby or people at the dog park. Friendships blossom. Sometimes, two strangers even meet and fall in love. I know, because it happened to me.

It was seven-thirty a.m., and I was outside with my foster dog, Sally, a black Labrador puppy I was raising for a guide dog organization. I'd just rolled out of bed. I was wearing sweatpants and a baggy T-shirt. My hair was standing out of my head, Medusa-like, in every direction. Sally had just stopped to take a poop when I heard footsteps approaching, and a deep voice said hello. I turned around to find a handsome man smiling at Sally and me. His name was Mike. He'd moved into my neighborhood in Los Altos while I'd been living in Santa Rosa, and even though I'd been back for more than a year, we'd never met. I blushed thinking about how Sally and I must look, me with my disheveled hair and slovenly clothes, Sally casually doing her business by my side.

Mike was unfazed and said he missed having a dog. He seemed

smart, funny, and kind. The conversation was brief, but I walked away feeling breathless and giddy. It took a few more chance encounters, when I was wearing more fashionable clothes and my hair was brushed, for a spark to ignite. When it did, Mike and I went on to share five laughter-filled and supportive years together, and he became one of the great loves of my life.

My "meet cute" (as Hollywood screenwriters call quirky first romantic encounters) is just one example of something that happens fairly often when we venture into public with our pets, according to research. When Australian researchers conducted a telephone survey of randomly selected residents in Perth, San Diego, Portland, and Nashville, they found that pet owners were significantly more likely to get to know people in their neighborhoods than those who didn't have companion animals. One woman in Nashville explained, "When we were first moving into the neighborhood some neighbors came over and noticed our cats and said if you need someone to watch your cats while you are away, we'll be happy to do it. Another neighbor has a couple of cats as well, and we initially got to know one another as we were watching the cats work things out among themselves." Another woman from San Diego said, "There's a path in our neighborhood that people walk along with their dogs. When you walk that path at the same time every day, you run into the same people and start conversations and make friends."

Indeed, in 40 percent of cases, the researchers found, participants said the acquaintances they met through their pets became *close* friends, who provided emotional and practical support—the type of person you'd call when you've just dropped your first child off at college or who shows up with ice cream and magazines after you've had surgery.

From a health perspective, the ramifications of that finding are profound. While loneliness can erode your emotional and physical well-being, the opposite is also true: People with more social contacts have higher day-to-day well-being and actually live longer, healthier lives. I love this study because it brings to light an underrecognized facet of our relationships with pets. They're more than just companions. They're social icebreakers, sledgehammering through our natural resistance to engaging with strangers and giving us a natural way to strike up a conversation. "Pets not only give you something to talk about and bond over, but studies show that people view others as friendlier and more approachable when they're with a pet," says Johnson. "And, often, when you start talking about your pets, you find other things you have in common."

Interactions that begin with a spontaneous comment like, "Your dog is so cute. What breed is he?" can evolve into, "Hey, should we go grab a cup of tea?" or "I have two tickets to the baseball game this weekend. Do you want to join me?" In measurable, tangible ways, pets can break down barriers that prevent us from knowing our neighbors, link individuals within communities, and pave the way for true friendships, and sometimes even love, to grow.

Pets Lure Us into the Magical Realm of Play

When Judy adopted Yuki, the little dog didn't simply relieve her loneliness. Just as good friends do, Yuki brightened Judy's world by adding a critical ingredient that many of us are missing: play. This underrated but ever-present aspect of sharing our homes with animals can actually fill an important need for all humans, not just those who are lonely, according to Stuart Brown, MD, founder of the National Institute for Play, a nonprofit whose goal is to expand the scientific knowledge of play and elevate its status in our culture—and our lives. "Play is energizing and enlivening," Dr. Brown told us. "It boosts your mood, reduces stress, and helps you feel more optimistic. It bolsters curiosity, perseverance, and a sense of mastery. For children, it's important in helping them understand the rules of social behavior. There are innumerable lessons embedded in what most of us still think of as a 'purposeless' activity. Research shows it's important for the well-being and survival of many animals, including humans."

Scientists can't fully explain the urge to play, though it seems to be encoded in our DNA, honed by 100 million years of evolution. Consider this: Nearly every species of mammal and many birds engage in some form of play. Ravens in Alaska are known to slide down steep, snow-covered roofs; when they reach the bottom, they go right back up to the top and do it again. Elephants like to slide, too—only they do it down muddy slopes, intentionally colliding with other pachyderms making their way up. (Elephant bowling!) "Domestic rats love to wrestle," says Dr. Brown. "Take away their playtime and they're more likely to be edgy, temperamental, and have a hard time getting along with their fellow rodents."

Dr. Brown became interested in the topic early in his career as a psychiatrist, while he was studying young homicidal males. After interviewing his study subjects, he realized their childhoods shared an important and hitherto unidentified trait: an absence of play. "The idea stuck with me," he says. "I realized by ignoring play we were missing a crucial element of what makes us healthy, socially adept humans." Since 1989, when he left his clinical practice, Dr. Brown has devoted himself full-time to studying the gleeful phenomenon in animals and humans.

As a result of his background, what he sees today troubles him. "We have a play deficit," he says. As work bleeds into home life thanks to email and cell phones, more and more of us view play as nonessential—a time-consuming luxury that, because it doesn't get us ahead professionally, we can no longer afford. "Adults' unstructured time has radically diminished, and children's outdoor playtime has decreased seventy-one percent in the last generation," he says. "That matters, because play is the crucible in which children's empathy is refined. As they play together and hear other children's contributions to the game, they come to understand different points of view. Play is necessary for the development of social awareness, cooperation, empathy, and fairness. That give-and-take is the basis of all relationships throughout our lives."

In other words, goofing around is good for us. And animals,

by their very nature, bring out this primal urge that lives inside of people. "Humans and animals communicate play signals clearly," Dr. Brown says. "When a dog does a play bow, most of us don't need someone to tell us what that means. When we accept the invitation and join an animal in play, it makes us both feel better." Such play communication across species lines is common, he adds. "Dogs and polar bears play, as do magpies and bears. There's a language of play that transcends speech and species."

Pets allow us to be silly. They encourage us to be uncool. They push us to run and throw Frisbees and immerse ourselves in nature—and to *appreciate* it once we're there.

Nearly every person who submitted a mutual rescue story mentioned that their adopted animal made them laugh. My cat Wilbur once unzipped a friend's purse, pulled out a scone he smelled inside, and ate it. Langley, another of my former cats, used to routinely hide behind plants and jump out to surprise me—a game so clearly intended to make me shriek that I'm convinced felines have a wonderful, if slightly devious, sense of humor.

The gifts of play are clear: Play helps us enter a world where, for a moment or two, or even an hour or a day, we're insulated from the realities of life. Inside that alternate universe, our egos fall away, and we're much more likely to engage with the present moment like animals do: less encumbered by rational thought and more able to experience pure, frivolous pleasure. After dangling yarn for a feisty cat or throwing a slobbery tennis ball for a dog, we re-enter our regular lives feeling lighter, calmer, and more energized—and often chuckling with delight at how our animals help us let go of the demanding reins of adulthood and feel free.

While scientists speculate that early humans bonded with dogs and cats millennia ago because they helped with hunting and cleared homes of rodents, I like to think the reason our forebears became so attached to these wild creatures is because animals made life more entertaining—and a lot more fun.

"Even at my lowest point, Ishy could make me smile," says Lis.

"And once my boyfriend and I moved in with each other, he learned to love her, too. Watching her and playing with her was a big focus of our relationship. She was just happy to be with us, and we were happy to be with her."

For Judy, who lives alone, Yuki's playfulness was eye-opening—and life-changing. "Her presence has made my life more fun than it's been in years. One of our favorite games is tag. When I stand in my kitchen with the island between us, I'll give her a certain look and begin to stoop down. She knows that's the signal to chase me around the island. When she 'tags' me with her paws, she gets a treat," says Judy. "Yuki brought love and laughter and fun back into my world. She's the best companion I could have asked for at this stage in my life. Our connection is magical. Yuki didn't just rescue me from my solitude. She brought an element of lightheartedness that I didn't even know I was missing."

7

Overcoming Illness and Injury

The Role of Pets in Persevering Through
Physical Challenges

It was June 8, 2013, the day of the Belmont Stakes, the third jewel in the Triple Crown of Thoroughbred Racing. Tracy Campion, a writer and avid equestrian in Kirkland, Washington, had just listened to the race on the radio when she went into the arena to ride her own horse, Beau. Shortly after she got into the saddle, Beau spooked and began to buck. "He could hear, but not see, horses running around outside—so it scared him," she recalls. "Beau was a sweet, sensitive guy. He had never bucked before, so I hung on and gripped his body with my legs and feet, hoping it would pass." Instead, he bucked again. And again. What Tracy didn't realize: She'd forgotten to take the spurs off her boots—something she always did before riding her reactive horse—so every time she tightened her grip on his body, she unknowingly spurred him, scaring him more. "He eventually did this violent spin that catapulted me out of the saddle and high into the air like a rag doll."

When Tracy landed, she hit the ground *hard*. A lifelong horse-woman, she'd been thrown a number of times over the years, but she'd never experienced anything like this. The impact knocked the wind out of her. As scary, she could hear Beau careening around the arena. She tried to scramble to her feet, terrified he might accidentally stomp her. That's when she realized she couldn't move her legs. She finally regained her breath and screamed for help. A friend came running and called 911.

Although it took five days to get a proper diagnosis, imaging tests eventually revealed that Tracy had shattered both the right and left sides of her pelvis and broken her sacrum, a large, triangular bone at the base of the spine. "The pain was excruciating," she says. "I couldn't even sit up without help. Every time I moved, my pelvis felt like a bicycle wheel with playing cards in its spokes. I was broken, in every sense of the word."

Confined to a wheelchair for months, alternately dazed with pain or battling nausea from the medication she took to alleviate it, Tracy felt like a stranger to herself. Prior to the accident, she'd put in long days as a writer—and hiked and ridden her horses in her off hours. Now she couldn't walk. She couldn't work. She could barely sleep or eat. She was so incapacitated she had to ask her husband to help her into the shower. "It was terrible feeling so helpless," she says. "I'd go ten days without a shower, because I hated asking for help—but having dirty hair made me feel even worse about myself."

By September, she was finally given the green light to start the grueling process of physical therapy. "I had to completely relearn to walk, so it was painful and humbling—my body was so stiff and rigid I had to try to remember how to bend my knees—but at least I was doing something," she says.

For the next year, she pushed herself to get back to normal. She progressed from a wheelchair to walking with crutches, but her noticeable limp made her self-conscious about being out in public, and her lingering fatigue and pain limited her ability to work. "Normal" was still a long way off, and she could feel herself sinking into despair. Before the accident, she and her husband had been talking about getting a dog, but they were planning to wait until they bought a house. Looking for something to brighten her mood, she said to him, "Why not do it now?"

Not long before, in nearby Yakima, a sweet, eighteen-month-old black Lab mix had been hit by a car. Someone found him by the side of the road and took him to Seattle Humane, where they performed surgery, saving his life. When Tracy and her husband arrived at the shelter, he'd just been put up for adoption. "We walked inside, and in the very first kennel there was this black dog," Tracy recalls. "I'd had a black Lab as a kid, so whenever I envisioned the dog I wanted that's what I pictured. He looked like he had one leg tucked underneath him, but when he moved I saw that it was missing.

"I said to my husband, 'Does he have three legs?' and my husband said, 'Yes.' Then the dog looked at us, and I said, 'Does he have one eye?' and my husband said, 'Yes.' The shelter employee encouraged us to take our time and meet some other dogs, but when I turned away the black dog put his paw up on the glass. I took a deep breath and said to my husband, 'This is our dog,' and he said, 'I know.'"

Until that time, Tracy had been reluctant to go for walks because her limp made her self-conscious. But her new dog, Jack—his missing eye made him look like a pirate, so she named him after Captain Jack Sparrow from *Pirates of the Caribbean*—had different plans. His bouncy joy was undimmed by his missing limb. He pestered her until they went out for a walk several times every day. In public, Jack's enthusiasm was so contagious it eased Tracy's anxiety about her own disability. "He is a total extrovert. He doesn't care if he's missing a leg and an eye. He wants to say hi to everyone. He's just a super entertaining dog—so the focus was always more on him than me," she says.

Nearly a year after bringing Jack home, Tracy had become strong and fit. But she'd also suffered additional heartbreak. In the intervening months she and her husband had split up. "It was a rough year. Without Jack, I don't know what I would have done—but we made it through," she says.

On her birthday that year, she took Jack out for a walk, and he gamboled ahead, as usual. As she marveled at his lilting stride and breathtaking ability to disregard his afflictions, she was overcome by a wave of such joy she decided to join him. "I took off running. Jack looked at me with this unmistakable expression of amazement, and I just started to laugh. I couldn't believe I was running, either—and it actually felt *good*," she says. "When I adopted Jack I was drawn to him partly because I thought no one else would adopt him. I thought I was doing him a favor. I realized that day I had it all wrong. I'd been the one who needed help all along."

The Boundless Need for Physical Healing

Tracy is a strong woman—determined, capable, not easily daunted. Against her doctor's advice, she went to the stable four months after her accident and started riding again—before she was even able to walk without help. She was apprehensive—but she was more distressed by the idea of developing a full-blown fear of riding if she let too much time pass. So she forced herself to do it. She made good on the cliché: She got back on her horse. Even so, she had trouble mustering that same resourcefulness when it came to walking and rebuilding her strength. Like many—maybe even most—people who are physically broken, whether due to illness or injury, Tracy needed an extra push—something or someone to motivate and inspire her to put in the difficult, uncomfortable hours of effort it took to fully regain her mobility. Some people get that push from a physical therapist. Others hire a trainer or join a gym or do yoga or receive acupuncture. Tracy's push came in the form of an eager three-legged stray.

In the previous chapter we explained that canines can encourage people to exercise—and Jack undoubtedly did that for Tracy. But he is more than a fitness partner. He helped her cope more directly with her physical challenges, eased her anxiety about her lingering limp, and gave her the equilibrium to withstand the back-to-back traumas of injury and divorce. And she's just one of millions of ill and injured people around the world who have found they can rely on animal companions in ways they never would have imagined.

The history of healing with animals goes back thousands of years. There's evidence from the ninth century that the Flemish used animals to assist in treating disabled people. In 1830, the British charity commissioner recommended having animals on the grounds of mental institutions. And in the 1860s, the Germans used animals as part of the treatment for epilepsy. Today, dogs' and cats' unique abilities to provide practical support are becoming ever more widely recognized by the medical profession and codified into our culture, with the growth of therapy animals, service animals, and emotional support animals. As a result, we're rediscovering what Florence Nightingale, legendary nurse and early proponent of animal-assisted therapy, pointed out in her *Notes on Nursing* in 1859: "A small pet is often an excellent companion for the sick or long chronic cases, especially."

That's good news, considering the staggering numbers of people who could benefit. At least 117 million people in the United States are coping with some sort of chronic illness or condition (defined as a disease that lasts for three months or longer)—from stroke to arthritis to cancer. For roughly 40 million of them, the problem is so severe it limits their ability to participate in their usual activities. In other words, their lives are diminished in meaningful ways.

More than 35 million people are hospitalized in the United States every year, and a growing number of hospitals across the country have incorporated animal-assisted therapy, animal-assisted activities, or pet visitations into their programs. A 2014 review of randomized controlled trials on therapy dogs in hospitals concluded that animal-assisted interventions may improve the quality of life for cancer patients and others with chronic or terminal illnesses and could improve self-reported outcomes in a variety of other conditions. Studies have shown that the presence of animals can also reduce pain and stress and motivate people to be more active, helping them push harder and longer in physical therapy.

At the same time, 2.8 million people who wind up in the hospital are there with traumatic injuries, and depending on the extent of the damage, recovery can take weeks, months, or sometimes even years. While our bodies possess a surprising capacity to bounce back, some injuries and illnesses don't just shatter bones or invade organs, they shatter lives, leaving the afflicted person to weave the tattered pieces of their existence back together. The more pervasive the damage, the tougher that can be. When Australian researchers followed two hundred people with serious injuries for six months, they found that slightly more than half suffered from depression and anxiety at some point—and those who'd sustained wounds severe enough to be admitted to the intensive care unit were at the highest risk. A Norwegian study of 194 ICU patients found that only 55 percent had returned to work a year later.

Cats can't cure cancer and dogs can't treat seizures, but they can, in many cases, improve chronically ill or injured people's ability to function, keep them safe, ease their suffering, and allow them to participate more fully in life—and the list of conditions animals might be able to help with just keeps growing, from post-op recovery to seizure disorders and Parkinson's to cancer, diabetes, and AIDS.

The specific roles that animals play are just as diverse. Nurse. Helpmate. Protector. Fitness partner. Cheerleader. Emotional support. Guardian. Friend. Like Tracy's dog, Jack, many of the animals aren't officially registered or trained to offer support. They're just pets—often rescue pets, who have endured their share of suffering. But they're able to give people the support they need to endure punishing treatments, push through the pain, and fight fiercely to return to themselves and the full richness of life.

"Having a pet motivates hospitalized patients to do what's needed to get well so they can return home—and once they're home, their pets reduce stress and help them stay engaged and active, which can help with healing," Edward Creagan, MD, told us. A professor of medical oncology at the Mayo Clinic School of Medicine, Dr. Creagan received the Distinguished Mayo Clinician award—Mayo Clinic's highest honor—and is a fellow of the American Academy of Hospice and Palliative Medicine. He and his wife also have three rescue animals at home—two cats and a golden retriever. "Research has shown that people with pets take fewer medications and visit the doctor less often, and I'm not surprised, given my experience with animals, personally and professionally. Long ago I noticed the effect pets had on my hospitalized patients with cancer. People are transformed when they talk about their cats and dogs. The subject brings a sense of humanity into a cold, gray, clinical hospital environment. I always write down the name of patients' pets when I take a medical history. Animals have a reproducible, restorative healing power that medical professionals would be wise to tap into."

The "100 Percent Pure-Bred Mutt" Who Helps One Woman Function

In 2010, Nora Delaney, of San Jose, California, was recovering from her eleventh hip surgery in eight years—the result of congenital arthritis that had plagued her since birth. She and her husband had been talking about getting a dog for a couple of years, and, as she sat in her wheelchair, she decided the time had come. "We hoped to be able to train a dog to do things for me that I couldn't do—but I figured at the very least a dog would be good company while I healed," says the operations director at a tech firm.

They went online and found a four-month-old puppy that had been rescued, along with his two brothers, from an industrial section of Bakersfield and taken to Animal Friends Rescue Project in Pacific Grove, not far from the Delaneys' home. The online listing said the dog was a dachshund–cocker spaniel mix. "He was just eleven pounds and looked like a mini golden retriever," says Nora.

When Nora and her husband went to the shelter, an employee let the puppy out of his kennel to meet the couple. "He licked my husband's toes, then ran to the toy bin, grabbed a rubber chicken, and put it at my feet, his tail going a million miles an hour," she recalls. "We took him out for a short walk to make sure he wouldn't get underfoot when I was using crutches, and he was perfect. He maintained a safe perimeter around me. He seemed to know instinctively not to get too close."

The Delaneys named their wriggly new charge Max and began reading books and watching videos about dog training so Nora's husband could teach the energetic pup to do things for her. Nora loved watching Max learn, but because she wasn't the one doing the training, she didn't feel an intense connection to their new dog. That all changed one day about two months after they brought Max home. "My husband wasn't home, so it was just Maxie and me—and he got his front paw caught in his training harness," she recalls. "The harder he struggled to free himself, the more the harness tightened around his neck. I wheeled my chair as close to Max as I could get, and told him to come, but he wouldn't do it. I was frantic, because I thought he was going to strangle himself. I was just about to throw myself on the floor, which would have set my healing back, but I said one more time, 'Max! Come!' He recognized my desperation. So he scooched toward me, got himself up onto his hind legs, and put his head and torso on my lap so I could remove the harness. When I finally got him disentangled, I looked at him and he looked at me and we just connected. It was like we realized we could trust each other. Our lives were never the same."

After that experience, Max seemed to understand that there were lots of things he could do that Nora couldn't—and he quickly picked up how to help. "Within a few weeks he was able to fetch my cell phone and bring me his bowl at mealtime and put away his own toys and bring me his leash," Nora says. "Once I was able to walk again, I still could only bend ninety degrees at the waist, and that's true to this day. So Max got in the habit of following me around the house. If I drop something he picks it up. I don't even have to say anything anymore. He just picks up Kleenex or lipstick or whatever and follows me until I get somewhere I can sit down. Then he gives it to me."

When they're out of the house, Max helps her as well. "He'll fetch items off low shelves at Home Depot, and when we're at the farmer's market he'll grab every bag of produce I buy and take it to my husband so I don't have to carry it. He's so cute and smart that people are constantly asking me what breed he is, and I tell them he's one hundred percent pure-bred American mutt. He's the best ambassador for rescue animals. Everyone is amazed at what he can do—but no one more than me. I had no idea how much his companionship and his ability to know what I need would improve my life."

He also brings her comfort. "When I'm in pain he'll lie down next to me. He's so empathetic, he even winces and cries sometimes. And he watches me constantly. It's the funniest thing. He just stares at me. It's like he's always trying to figure out what I want. He knows his job is to help me, and he takes it seriously. When you can't walk properly, you start to feel very different from everyone else, but Max doesn't treat me like I'm different. He treats me like I'm special. It's quite wonderful. Together, he and I are a force to be reckoned with."

The Deeply Rooted Reason Dogs Are So Helpful

Every single time I see a guide dog walking down the street with its sight-impaired owner, vigilantly avoiding obstacles and stopping at crosswalks, I marvel at canines' capacity to work in collaboration with humans. I mean, really. We don't speak the same language. We don't share the same ability to reason and think. We ambulate differently and eat differently and show affection differently. Why would a dog be willing to subjugate impulses to sniff and pee and chase squirrels in order to provide assistance to a person who can't see?

Turns out I'm not the only one who is enthralled by that question. The phenomenon of human-animal cooperation has captured the interest of a number of scientists around the world, and their research is beginning to trace the origins and track the biological basis of dogs' uncanny abilities.

"Dogs are fascinating creatures, because they have so thoroughly adapted to living with humans. The question that intrigues me is where their unusual ability to become part of our lives comes from," Zsofia Viranyi told us, "and in order to answer that question you need to study their ancient relatives, wolves." Viranyi cofounded Austria's Wolf Science Center with Friederike Range and Kurt Kotrschal, whose research we highlighted in Chapter 1, and her work is helping shed light on the unaccountable mystery of human-canine cooperation.

For years, researchers have believed that when the least aggressive wolves began living alongside humans, they evolved to become more cooperative creatures, because the more amenable animals were the ones most likely to survive long enough to pass along their genes. And that's true, says Viranyi—to an extent. Based on recent research at the Wolf Science Center, she and her colleagues have developed what they call the canine cooperation hypothesis—essentially that when early wolves started interacting with humans more than 30,000 years ago, the animals were *already* extremely social, cooperative creatures.

"Researchers have always portrayed wolves as aggressive, but as we've watched our wolf packs over the years a very different picture has emerged," she says. "Wolves are highly affiliated animals. The mother and father and children synchronize their shared behaviors. They live together and play together and hunt together and groom each other. And when we humans work with them, they're able to understand and respond to our communication in much the same way dogs do."

When wolves began living with humans, they were already oriented toward cooperative behavior—and in the intervening millennia, canines have become even more attentive to us and invested in our mutual care, elevating their ability to collaborate to an art form. For instance, dogs are more docile than wolves and thus more responsive to behavioral inhibition: A sharp "No!" is usually enough to prevent your pet from grabbing food from the table, for instance. "Wolves will just go ahead and take the food," says

Viranyi. "By evolving alongside early humans, dogs developed the ability to inhibit their impulses."

Today, their willingness to submit to our directives—come, sit, stay, heel, fetch—forms the cornerstone of their utility as therapy and service animals. Service dogs are particularly gifted at taking direction. These animals, recognized by the government's American with Disabilities Act, receive hours of training to learn to be the eyes and ears for people with physical disabilities, like visual or hearing impairment, diabetes or seizures or a severe emotional challenge like PTSD. Researchers at Emory University conducted brain imaging tests where they trained dogs to hold still in an fMRI machine (a more sophisticated type of MRI that allows doctors to see not only the brain's structure but also identify the regions with increased blood flow, a sign of brain activity). The studies revealed that those who perform best as service dogs have greater activity in their caudate, a C-shaped region deep within each of the brain's hemispheres, that plays a vital role in learning and storing and processing memories and is important to the development of language and communication.

In addition, dogs are more dependent on humans than wolves— and the more dependent animals are, the more attached they're likely to be to their owners. When Max follows Nora around the house picking up after her, or Jack lies by Tracy's side while she's working, the humans benefit—but the dogs have a stake in whether their people are okay, too. "Dogs know they're dependent on us for their food and safety, so they keep an eye on us to make sure we're okay," Viranyi says. "Their natural inclination to watch us makes them highly suitable as service animals. In fact, the dogs that make the best partners for people with epileptic seizures, for instance, are highly dependent and develop a strong attachment to their owners."

Through millennia of domestication, we've actually transformed canines, to the extent that it's possible, into four-legged facsimiles of ourselves, adds Juliane Kaminski, PhD, a senior lecturer in the department of psychology at the University of Portsmouth, who began studying dogs as a way to gain a better understanding of human cognition. Her research has shown, for instance, that many dogs can learn words—and an unusual handful have better vocabularies than the average toddler. For instance, Kaminski conducted a study with Rico, a border collie, who knew the names of two hundred objects. He held the record until 2010, when psychologists from Wolford College in Spartanburg, South Carolina, announced they had taught Chaser, another border collie, the names of 1,022 toys. (It took sixteen plastic tubs to hold all of them.)

Whether dogs actually understand what we want, much less why we want it, remains an open question, says Kaminski. What *is* clear, she says, is that dogs are motivated to help people. "They're keen to interact and bond with us, and they're constantly trying to figure out what we want," she says. "There's no other animal on the planet that's as good at interpreting our communicative behavior—not even chimpanzees, who are much closer to us genetically.

"Domestication helped dogs tune into us in this remarkable way and opened this channel where information coming from us became incredibly relevant to them," she says. "Our interspecies communication is really good. Regardless of what they understand about us, they can be wonderful family members and helpers. They understand what we want them to do, even if they don't understand why."

A Laid-Back Cat Comforts People in the ICU

When Jennifer Morris's five-year-old daughter, Isa, had a Monday off school in November 2010, Morris decided to take her to San Francisco Animal Care and Control to visit the cats. "We both love cats, and our beloved cat had died a week earlier, so we were both sad," Jennifer says. As they walked around the facility, one black cat kept meowing. And meowing. I was looking at the other animals, but my daughter came up to me and said, 'I want the black-and-white kitty. I love him.'"

A shelter employee let them into the caged area where the

talkative cat was pacing around, and the second they were inside, the cat made a beeline for Isa. "He was totally taken with her—rubbing against her legs, meowing. She was so excited. I hadn't intended to adopt a cat that day, but I figured what the heck? He seemed great, and he made Isa happy," she says.

The cat had been found in a starving feral colony in downtown San Francisco. When Animal Control picked him up, they housed him in the part of the shelter with the other feral cats—but quickly realized that wasn't where he belonged. The black-and-white feline wasn't just friendly to people. He *loved* them. And everyone loved him in return, including Jennifer and Isa. Two days later, they went to pick up their new cat, who looked so dapper with his tuxedo-like black-and-white markings that they named him Duke Ellington.

On the way home from the shelter, Jennifer warned Isa that Duke would probably disappear in the house for a couple of days until he had time to get used to his new surroundings. She couldn't have been more wrong. "When we got home, he strutted around like he owned the place. He found the litter box. He found the scratching post. He walked around like he was the boss," recalls Jennifer. Later that night, when her boyfriend arrived, the first one to greet him at the door was Duke Ellington.

"At that moment I realized this cat was special," she says. "I work as an analyst at the University of California at San Francisco's School of Nursing, and I thought he'd make a good therapy cat." She was busy with work, so she didn't pursue it right away. But two years later, she went to San Francisco SPCA's therapy-animal orientation and had Duke evaluated to see if he met the criteria for a therapy animal. "There was this big group of people there to test him, and Duke loved it. He loved being the center of attention."

Because Jennifer works at UCSF, she talked to the coordinator of the therapy animal program and got Duke set up in the rotation in the intensive care unit. Cats are still fairly uncommon as therapy animals. Of the 11,000 pets registered with Pet Partners, one of the largest and most highly regarded organizations that registers therapy animals in the United States, just 2 percent are cats—which is a shame, says Dr. Creagan, because, like dogs, laid-back and friendly cats can offer comfort and support to patients. Personality matters more than species—or pedigree. Indeed, *many* of Pet Partners' therapy animals are rescues. "We see over and over again that shelter animals can make wonderful therapy animals. When someone in the hospital reaches over to pet a dog, a struggling student reads with confidence to a rabbit, or a nursing home resident with dementia recalls a cat they once loved while one is resting comfortably by their side, it makes no difference if that animal came through a shelter. The benefits from the human-animal bond are still profound," said Annie Peters, CEO of Pet Partners.

Peters's comments affirm something those of us in the rescue community witness every day: Having known suffering and rejection themselves, many shelter animals appear to have gained a sense of wisdom, for lack of a better word, born of personal hardship and pain. As a result, the benefits of animal therapy can be even *more* profound when the creature in question is a rescue, because *two* beings are transformed: A human receives healing and hope, and an animal that has so much more to give to the world is granted redemption.

Not all ICUs allow therapy animals—but a 2018 editorial in the medical journal *Critical Care* by a team of health care professionals from Johns Hopkins School of Medicine hypothesized that pet visits could be a way to address common heartbreaking issues that crop up in patients who are in critical condition. ICU patients, for instance, often require feeding tubes, catheters, mechanical ventilators to help them breathe, and a variety of other interventions that are not only frightening and uncomfortable but also dehumanizing and demoralizing. As a result of the stress, medication, and inactivity, up to 80 percent of ICU patients develop delirium—they're confused, disoriented, and may hallucinate. "Through creating humanized

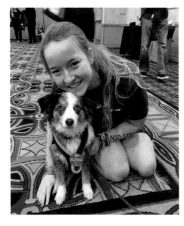

Grace Briden with rescue therapy dog, Karma (*Marni Bellavia Photography*)

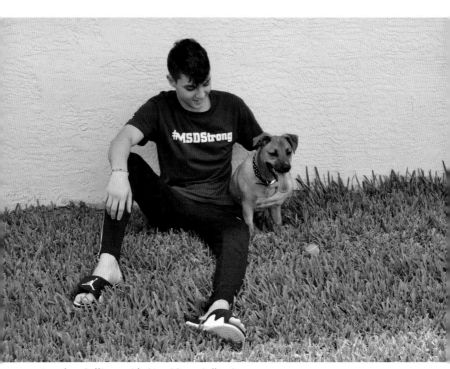

Jonathan Sullivan with Ajax (*Gerry Sullivan*)

View additional photos at book.MutualRescue.org/photos

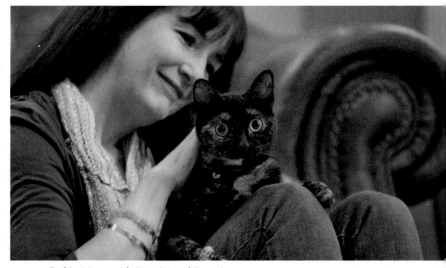

Robin Myers with Liza *(Mutual Rescue)*

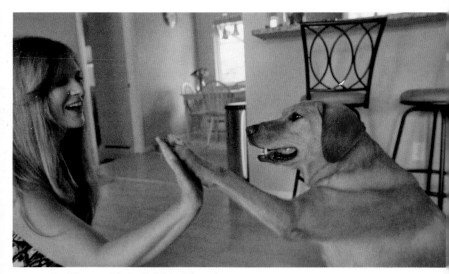

Jessi Burns with Andi *(Mutual Rescue)*

View additional photos at book.MutualRescue.org/photos

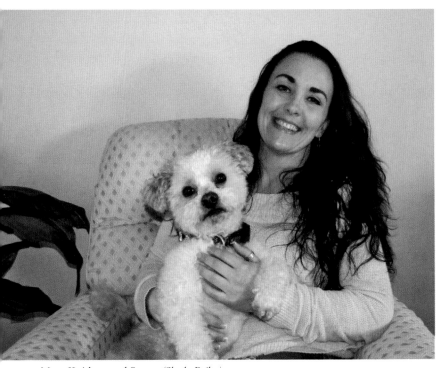

Mary Kniskern and Sonny *(Sharla Bailey)*

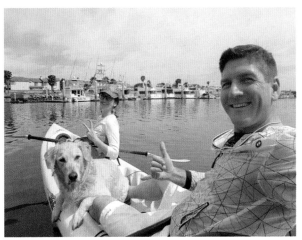

Matt Earnest and his sister Kelly with Samson *(El Disco)*

View additional photos at book.MutualRescue.org/photos

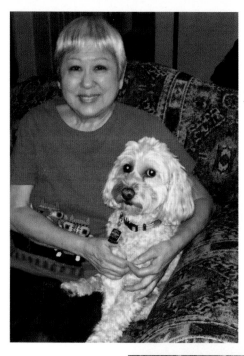

Judy Torigoe with Yuki
(Lisa Schmidt)

Tracy Campion with Jack
(Sarah Bous-Leslie)

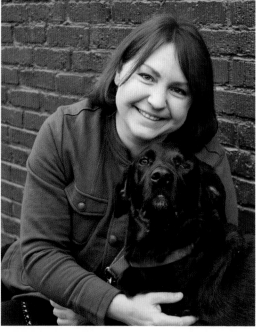

View additional photos at book.MutualRescue.org/photos

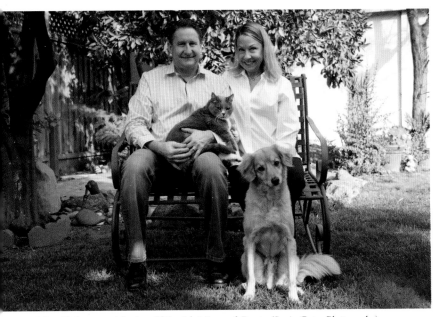

Nora Delaney and husband JB with Max and Boots *(Sonia Gates Photography)*

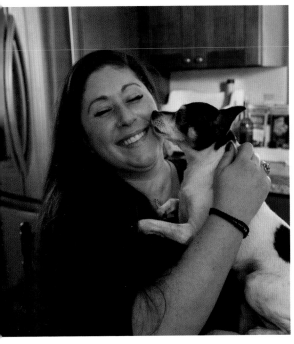

Sarah Coletti and Domino
(Mutual Rescue)

View additional photos at book.MutualRescue.org/photos

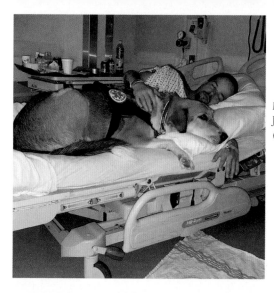

Meatball visiting
Joe McCarty in the hospital
(*Joe and Kim McCarty*)

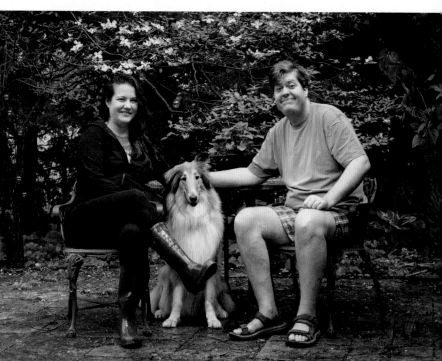

Alexis Hurley and Drew Hurley with Guinness *(Eric Limon)*

View additional photos at book.MutualRescue.org/photos

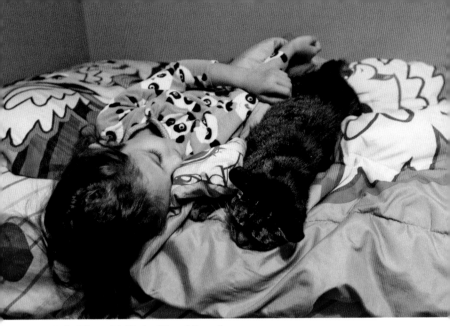

Jade Allen with Trubs *(Mutual Rescue)*

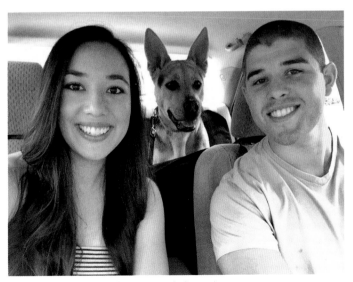

Kim and Brian Rose with Lana *(Kimberly Rose)*

View additional photos at book.MutualRescue.org/photos

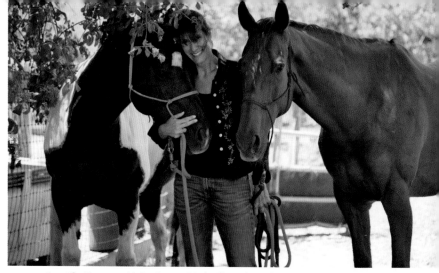

Jennifer Fenton with her horses Nashville and Frankie *(Molly Hansen Photography)*

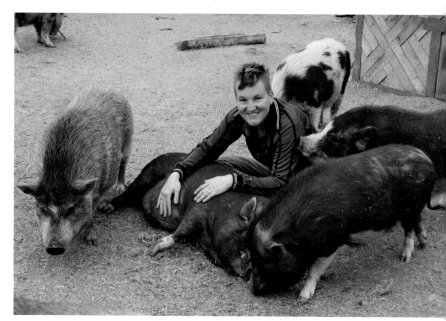

Erin Brinkley-Burgardt with Pippy, Boris, Chopper, Pumba, and Harley
(Erin Brinkley-Burgardt)

View additional photos at book.MutualRescue.org/photos

ICU environments and implementing non-pharmacological interventions, patients no longer must wait for hospital discharge before they begin to live again," the authors wrote. "Non-pharmacological intervention programs, such as animal-assisted interventions, may reduce suffering and help patients take an active role in their recovery."

During her monthly visits to the ICU with Duke, Jennifer saw that idea become a reality. On the day of Duke's scheduled rounds, she'd drive home at lunchtime, pick him up, and bring him back to the hospital, where she'd wheel him around the ICU on a medical cart (she learned early on that Duke prefers being up high so he can see what's going on) to visit patients for an hour or two.

"It was incredible to see the impact he had," says Jennifer. "Being in the ICU is traumatic physically and emotionally. There's not a lot of joy in a place like that. But when Duke would come in the room, patients would light up. Seeing someone smile even though life had given them a whole bunch of lemons is really wonderful."

Matt Aldrich, MD, is the medical director of critical care medicine at UCSF and works with the Society of Critical Care Medicine to address the problems that often beset patients as a result of being in the ICU. He told us, "We've made a lot of progress with helping patients survive their illnesses, and now we're focusing on how to change the ICU experience to give them the best foundation for a healthy life once they're home. We're trying to get patients up and moving and use less sedation and keep them on a regular sleep-wake cycle. And part of that effort is creating opportunities for kindness and connection throughout the day. That's where animal visits come in. For people who find meaning in their relationships with animals—and many people do—a visit with a cat or dog can be calming and might even motivate them to engage in physical therapy. The presence of an animal can also counteract some of the loss of comfort and dignity you experience in the ICU. That's the type of intervention we want more ICUs to move toward."

Pets Help Patients Through Treatment and Recovery

In addition to the millions of sick people inside hospitals, there are many millions more outside, living at home and trying to grapple with serious illnesses on their own. They often struggle with depression, fear, and pain. But having an animal to care for can prevent them from sinking into apathy and help them, slowly and incrementally, move forward.

Take Finnegan Dowling. As a nineteen-year-old college student living 3,000 miles away from her family, she was diagnosed with Hodgkin's disease, a type of lymphatic cancer. She could have gone home to live with her parents in Connecticut, but she had a life in Olympia, Washington—and Seamus, a big yellow Lab–shar-pei mix she'd adopted from Joint Animal Services in Thurston County the year before. By the time Finn adopted him at eighteen months, Seamus had been returned to the shelter by two different owners because he was such a handful.

"The first time I put him in the back seat of my Volkswagen Beetle he shredded the entire thing. The stuffing got down in the engine and the engine caught fire," she says. "Fortunately, all he needed was regular exercise and to grow up a little. He turned into a fantastic dog." After her diagnosis, she learned just how wonderful he could be. During chemo she lost her hair and became jaundiced. "I'm five foot nine, and my weight dropped to ninety-two pounds, so I looked like a yellow death-cicle," she says. "It was difficult to deal with people's reactions. Their pity. Their awkwardness. College kids don't know what to say. So I retreated to the Airstream trailer where Seamus and I were living."

No matter how isolated she was, she couldn't give up. Seamus needed to be cared for. "On days when everything felt like despair wrapped in a thick coat of nausea, there was Sea with his tennis ball. On days I couldn't do more than let him in and out, he'd lie next to me on my bed, his warm body pressed against my leg like an anchor holding me to a world that felt farther away by the day." Chemo and radiation took more than a year, and Seamus was there through it all. Afterward, he was a bridge back to her friends—and her life. Finnegan is forty-three now and handles social media for Mutual Rescue. "I've worked on and off in animal welfare my whole life, partly thanks to Sea," she says. "I see him in every rescue dog, every day. When I was barely hanging on, he robbed me of the option of giving up. He robbed me of the option of staying in bed all day. He had no pity for me. Just pure, unadulterated love. His faith in me got me through."

Pets force us to stay engaged. They keep us tethered to life. They give us a reason to stay tethered. And they make us *happy* to be alive. "Before I adopted Jack, I spent hours sitting in a chair looking out the window at life passing me by," says Tracy Campion. "I had a lot of self-doubt and sadness. There were days I wondered if I'd ever feel like myself again. Jack turned all that around. Adopting a disabled dog helped me accept my own impairments. His missing leg is like a secret superpower. It makes him even more adorable. Watching him embrace life so fully showed me that I had a choice: Let my physical challenges define me or move past them and redefine myself."

When we initially hear about a three-legged dog in need of adoption or a dog that's been rejected by three different owners like Seamus, it's natural to focus on their imperfections and the things they lack—or the extra effort their care might require. But after witnessing thousands of people, many of whom are suffering physically, adopt pets with special needs, I know one thing for certain: Imperfect adoptees have something extraordinary to offer broken humans. Pets with problems of their own make us feel less alone in our infirmity, show us how to unflinchingly face fragility, and give us the opportunity to practice compassion—toward both our perfectly imperfect pets and ourselves. What may look at first like cracks are the vulnerable places where kindness and empathy—and ultimately love—can flourish.

8

Recovering from Addiction

The Stabilizing Power of Furry Acceptance

Gemma Hunt was six when her mom moved out, leaving her and her half brother and half sister with her dad, who had a hair-trigger temper. After her mom took her back two years later, the family moved frequently throughout central England, and Gemma, a shy kid and one of the few children of color in their mostly white neighborhoods, struggled to make friends. Their family dog, Tasha, a big, protective German shepherd, was Gemma's sole refuge and source of stability. "Tasha was my best friend," Gemma, now thirty-five, recalls. "We spent hours together. In some ways, she was like my mum. When I was young, she was really my only link to the outside world."

At age thirteen, Gemma discovered alcohol and, along with it, a group of hard-partying friends. But Tasha was still her touchstone. When the dog died two years later, Gemma's anguish over losing her best friend and closest ally pushed her deeper into substance use. "To cope with my pain and loneliness I'd go out and party so hard that I'd black out, and the next morning I wouldn't remember anything that happened," she says.

By her early twenties, hardly a day went by when she wasn't drunk. "I'd have a drink first thing in the morning, and it continued from there. My life was a shambles. I was living with a man I didn't particularly like, and I was working as an erotic dancer. I was constantly angry and felt sorry for myself. I saw myself as a victim of my circumstances who had no control over her own life," she says. On a whim one day, the couple went to the Bath Cats and Dogs Home, where they met Prince, a skinny, quiet boxer. "The minute we got him home we realized he was aggressive and dominant," Gemma recalls. "My energy was weak, and Prince sensed that, so he'd growl anytime I came near him. One day he went after me, and I had to lock myself in the kitchen. Needless to say, I had no real fondness for him."

Gemma moved out not long after. When she went back to get some of her things a week later, the house was empty—no clothes, no furniture, no Prince. "I didn't know what had happened to the dog, and I was devastated. I hadn't had a good relationship with Prince, but I was worried about him. I tried to find out where he was, but I couldn't get any information."

To cope with her sadness, she went back to the shelter with a friend to volunteer to walk the dogs, and someone who worked there told her they had recently received a stray boxer. "Before I even saw him I shouted, 'Prince!' and up popped his head. I was so happy to see that he was okay I took him home the next day," she says. "He was still dominant, but I wasn't scared of him anymore. Because I'd made the choice to take him on, I knew I needed to figure out how to handle him. One day when he growled and lunged at me, I stood my ground and told him firmly, 'No.' He looked at me for a moment, then rolled onto his back. After that, our bond solidified. There was nothing we didn't do together."

Gemma was still partying, but she began to curtail her time away from home so she could take better care of Prince, and she started focusing more of her attention on his needs. She bought him healthy food to help him gain weight. She worked with him for hours to rein in his aggressive behavior. She took him out for walks to get him better socialized. "We both loved the fresh air, so I got us each a backpack, and we'd walk for ten or fifteen miles at a time," she says.

Prince was becoming better behaved by the day, but Gemma's demons weren't as easy to tame. "I had trouble controlling my temper. If I dropped a spoon on the floor, for instance, I'd start smashing things and swearing at myself, because that's how my dad reacted to minor mishaps when I was a kid," she says. "But I noticed that every time I went mental, Prince did, too."

Early one morning, she stumbled in after a night of heavy partying and broke down. Sad, lonely, and disgusted by her own behavior, she was doubled over sobbing, when, out of nowhere, Prince started having a seizure. "It was terrifying. Seeing him in pain made me forget my problems. I held his shaking body and tried to calm him by talking quietly to him and telling him I loved him. All the while, I had this terrible feeling that his behavior was mimicking mine—like my chaotic emotions had caused the seizure—and I felt incredibly ashamed," she says. "I didn't want him to be unhappy. I knew I needed to try to get a grip on myself, if not for my own sake, for his."

It didn't happen overnight, but slowly, by taking care of Prince, she began taking better care of herself. She cut back on drinking and stopped erotic dancing and started getting more work in music videos and modeling. Then a mutual friend introduced her to Darren. "He was a kind, smart, stable guy in the military, and Prince loved him the first time he met him—which is saying something, because Prince wasn't crazy about men," she says.

They'd been dating only a few weeks when Darren told Gemma he didn't like her when she was drunk. "I realized that was the same thing Prince had been trying to tell me time after time in his own way," she says. "I knew I was facing a choice: Keep drinking and ruin my relationships with Darren and Prince, or give it up. From the time I was young, I'd been using alcohol as a way to escape my unhappiness. Drinking was a sign of my sense of hopelessness. I didn't care if I lived or died. But now I did care. I had a dog and a man who loved me unconditionally. I was happy—maybe for the first time ever. That was seven years ago. I've barely had a glass of wine since. I really can't stand the smell or taste of alcohol anymore. I embraced a life of love instead."

The Scary Scope of Addiction

In late 2017, a startling phrase from the news caught my attention: *deaths of despair*. It was referring to research by a pair of Princeton professors, who found that while mortality rates among people in midlife around the world continue to drop, the United States has experienced a troubling counter-trend. Since the 1990s, death rates in people in middle age (especially white, middle-class people) have actually steadily *risen*.

The researchers attributed that grim finding to two main factors: a slowdown in medical progress against cancer and heart disease, the two largest killers in middle age, and a rise in the number of "deaths of despair"—mortality related to drugs, alcohol, and suicide—signs of a deep, cultural malaise that, the researchers speculated, is driven largely by a deterioration of economic stability and social well-being. Reading the news is often upsetting, but that particular story broke my heart. The sense of hopelessness that Gemma felt—the social isolation, alienation, and detachment from things that have always mattered (extended family, long-term careers, neighbors, and community)—is spreading, and can be deadly.

That alarming idea is backed up by plenty of data. Nearly 21 million people in the United States abuse alcohol or drugs, and 175 die every day of drug overdoses, a number that has climbed at an alarming pace. The rate of deadly overdoses from synthetic opioids (pain drugs like tramadol, fentanyl and fentanyl derivatives) rocketed 88 percent every year from 2013 to 2016, the most lethal on record. More than 63,600 lives were lost to drug overdoses in 2016, a number that's roughly equivalent to American losses in the Vietnam and Iraq wars combined.

Although drugs and alcohol are taking a notable toll on people in midlife, the problem usually begins far earlier. More than 90 percent of people with addictions began drinking or using illicit substances before they were eighteen—not surprising, since a number of experts believe that the illness stems, at least in part, from early trauma, family conflict, and a lack of solid bonding with other people. When the humans in their life are a source of pain instead of comfort, teenagers, especially, may turn to substances for solace, and those with a genetic predisposition to addiction are more likely to get hooked.

Addiction, whether to opioids or alcohol, food or shopping, is a disease, like diabetes, but one of its risk factors is a lack of connection. And once substance use turns into abuse, it erodes ties with friends and family, limiting healthy bonding even further and leaving the user ever more isolated, with nothing but their drug of choice for consolation.

Only about 10 percent of people with substance-use disorders receive any type of treatment. However, studies show that about one in ten adults in the United States who have struggled with a drug or alcohol problem have actually managed to overcome it. In other words, there are healthy, thriving former substance abusers who have faced their demons and successfully turned their lives around, and their stories can give others hope.

Getting sober is challenging. There are myriad approaches, and what works for one person may not be effective for another. Moreover, the thinking on how best to help people steel themselves against their substance of choice and maintain their sobriety over a lifetime is still evolving—but one method that's gaining traction among experts is utilizing animals in treatment and recovery.

Bethany Ranes, PhD, a research scientist at the Hazelden Betty Ford Foundation's Butler Center for Research in Center City, Minnesota, recently reviewed the literature on using animal-assisted therapy in addiction treatment and was impressed enough with the results to recommend that the renowned treatment center expand its use of animals in its programs. "We went from two to seven therapy dogs throughout our campuses, and we're hoping to add more. The factor that persuaded us to bring more dogs on board was the literature finding that animals can help solidify the bond between therapist and patient. That's critically important. In a program like ours, it's that bond that really drives recovery."

Indeed, a new body of research shows that cats and dogs, who approach the world without judgment or blame, can often reach addicts when people can't. By doing so, animals can help restore people's confidence in their ability to connect with another living creature—an essential step in the process of overcoming addiction. Gemma is one moving example. Without Prince, she might have become one of millions of deaths of despair around the world. But she curbed her drinking so she could take better care of Prince, then stopped entirely because she was worried about the effect it was having on her relationships with both Prince and Darren.

And she's far from the only person whose motivation to change was driven in part by a four-legged partner. Throughout the recovery world, there is growing recognition that the structure and solace cats and dogs bring to addicts' lives can be one of the factors that helps ease the grip of their disease and offers them hope that a fresh start is possible.

How a Ten-Pound Pup Helped One Woman Kick Heroin

In her early twenties, Sarah Coletti of Peabody, Massachusetts, went to a well-regarded doctor in Boston to figure out what was causing the all-over body pain she was experiencing. She'd long struggled with aches and pains, but three car accidents exacerbated the problem. Eventually, the doctor diagnosed her with a connective tissue disorder, because her joints were hyper-mobile and prone to painfully dislocating.

To treat the pain, the doctor prescribed ibuprofen and Vicodin, an opioid-based painkiller, similar to heroin or methadone. When she was still suffering, he added Percocet, then OxyContin, both of which contain oxycodone, a type of opioid with a high potential for abuse. And that was in addition to the anti-anxiety drugs and muscle relaxants he also prescribed. "It got to the point where I couldn't work because I was taking so many meds," says Sarah, now thirty-five. "All those prescriptions should have been a red flag. But I trusted my doctor."

Eventually, her doctor lost his license because of his liberal prescribing habits, and the MD she saw next slashed her meds to a fraction of what they'd been. "I'd been taking a hundred forty milligrams of opioids a day, and the new doctor cut me back to ten milligrams, so I went into instant withdrawal. I'd never withdrawn from a drug before. Until then, I'd never even considered myself an addict. I was jumping out of my skin. It was brutal. I was just following my doctor's orders—and now I was addicted."

At the time, Sarah's hometown of Peabody was overrun with street drugs, especially opioids. One high school friend had already died of a heroin overdose, and a number of others were active users. So when Sarah lost access to her prescriptions, she followed the same route as many pain patients before her and since: She turned to "street pharmacists" for drugs. "OxyContin is expensive on the street. It would have cost me hundreds of dollars a day to get the amount I needed. But I could get heroin for five dollars. So that's what I did."

She started by sniffing little bits here and there, just to get by, but eventually—inevitably, she thinks now—she began injecting the drug. "I come from an upper middle class family. Heroin wasn't supposed to be part of my life. But there I was—a twenty-six-year-old IV drug user."

Sarah was far from alone. About 80 percent of heroin users today start with prescription opioids. And like most users, Sarah came face-to-face with the horrible reality of heroin addiction. She overdosed a number of times and saw dozens of friends OD as well. Some survived. Many didn't. She went through several rehabs, and several relapses. After getting out of her last treatment program in 2011, she moved from Massachusetts to Connecticut with her then-fiancé, a truck driver, and they decided to get a dog. "My fiancé was on the road all the time, and I was home alone. I had no nearby family and few friends. I was off heroin by then, but I was still abusing prescription muscle relaxants and anxiety meds, and I was deeply unhappy. I thought it might help me to have a companion," says Sarah.

Because they lived in a townhouse, Sarah and her fiancé could only have a small dog. Serendipitously, some friends said they knew of a family who had a two-year-old miniature rat terrier in need of a new home. "They sent us a photo. His name was Domino," Sarah recalls. "When we went to meet Domino, the poor thing was all skin and bones. He was frightened and shaking. He had a cat collar around his neck with a little bell on it, a cracked food bowl, and the cheapest kibble possible. The saddest thing was the life behind his eyes was gone. I knew that haunted look. I'd seen it in myself hundreds of times when I looked in the mirror. I couldn't wait to get him out of that situation."

For the first few days, the terrified pup was withdrawn and kept to himself, and although Sarah had no idea what might have happened to him, she was worried he might be so traumatized he'd never adjust to his new life. "Then about five days after we brought him home, he jumped up onto my lap and showered me with kisses. I think it took him that long to realize he wasn't going back to his prior home," says Sarah.

Not long after getting Domino, Sarah left her fiancé and returned to Peabody. Several months later, she was sitting at the kitchen table at a friend's house where she was housesitting. She'd been up all night smoking cigarette after cigarette and bingeing on her meds. The morning sun was streaming in the window. "I felt sort of dead inside. I remember thinking that if I don't get clean now I'm going to die. And then I looked down, and there was little Domino at my feet. He pawed at my leg and looked up at me, like, 'When can we go to bed?' It made me feel so bad. This little guy was depending on me. If I couldn't take care of myself, how dare I claim to be ready to take on a dog? I had a reason to stay clean and stay alive, and he was sitting at my feet.

"That was the turning point in my addiction," she adds. "When I first got clean I didn't feel comfortable around other humans. I was ashamed and felt that people were judging me. But dogs love you with reckless abandon, and having those positive feelings directed at me all the time was incredibly healing."

She found that she could cope with her pain better once Domino was in her life, too. And her experience isn't a one-off. In 2012, researchers from the University of Pittsburgh reported on a study in which they had a trained therapy dog visit patients in the waiting room of an outpatient clinic for fibromyalgia, a chronic pain condition. After just a ten-minute visit with the dog, more than a third of participants reported a significant drop in pain—an average of two points on an eleven-point scale.

"When I'm having a bad pain day, Domino will just lie next to me, and the feeling of his little body next to mine relaxes me and helps alleviate the pain," Sarah says. As important, Domino helped Sarah believe in herself and her future. "He gave me the courage to stick with a twelve-step sobriety program and the self-discipline to become a certified dog behaviorist. When I was using I didn't care if I lived or died. Now I do what I love and I love what I do. People who are addicted to opioids don't hear many stories of people getting clean. But I'm here to say that recovery is very much possible. And animals' compassion and empathy can help. Domino was able to do for me what no human could ever do. The only reason I'm here today, alive and thriving, is because of an unwanted ten-pound dog."

Why Animals Provide Hope for Addicts—and Those Who Treat Them

Research is beginning to show that Gemma's and Sarah's experiences aren't unusual. In 2016, the Canadian Centre on Substance Use and Addiction conducted its Canadian Life in Recovery survey, including, for the first time, questions about pets. In a general sense, the 855 respondents in recovery said they were doing well. Nearly 91 percent reported their quality of life in recovery was good or better than good; almost one-third said it was excellent. As hopeful, one section of the survey asked what informal supports participants used and found important to their recovery. Nearly 72 percent of respondents said they used pets as a source of support, and 88 percent said pets were a somewhat (32 percent) or very (60 percent) important aspect of recovery. Pets' importance ranked above other stay-well approaches like having a healthy nutrition or diet plan, engaging in art, poetry, or writing, and utilizing websites that support recovery.

"At its heart, addiction is about disconnection—from yourself or your traumatic past or the people who care about you in your life," explains Colleen Dell, PhD, a professor of sociology at the University of Saskatchewan, who specializes in animals and addiction treatment but wasn't directly involved in the survey. "There's so much stigma and shame with addiction it causes people to withdraw and to avoid reaching out for help. But animals don't judge or criticize or blame, so having an animal in therapy is an effective way to short-circuit the shame and stigma and get people to open up."

Adding a dog to a therapy session gives individuals recovering from addiction a being they can touch and hug, too—and that can be an important aspect of recovery. "Healthy touch can be extremely healing for people who've experienced trauma or who have anxiety—which includes the majority of people who struggle with substance abuse," Dell told us. "In my work, I've seen that the more hardened and disconnected a person is, the more benefit a therapy animal can have. And once an animal opens someone's heart, it creates a receptive space for building relationships with other people—therapists, support groups, or friends and family."

Reestablishing those connections can be an important factor in turning an addict away from substance use and toward recovery, agrees Bethany Ranes of Hazelden Betty Ford. After reviewing the literature on using animal-assisted therapy in the treatment of substance abuse, Ranes concluded that an animal can support and solidify the therapeutic alliance between therapist and patient.

"When there's a strong relationship between a therapist and client, relapse rates and re-admittance rates decline considerably. In the treatment realm, we're constantly trying to find ways to strengthen that bond—so it's thrilling and hopeful to find that animals are a viable way to do it."

Researchers from Kentucky compared a group of substance use patients who received animal-assisted therapy to those who didn't. They found that, regardless of the person—no matter their gender or whether they were pet owners or what types of substances they abused or what other mental health issues they were dealing with—addicts who went through the animal-assisted treatment program felt far more positively about their relationship with their therapist.

Dogs are integrated more often in treatment, but cats can be profoundly helpful, too—sometimes more so, according to Linda Chassman, PhD, cofounder and executive director of Animal Assisted Therapy Programs of Colorado—especially for patients who are having problems with social skills or who have anxiety or difficulty communicating with family and friends. "Dogs tolerate all kinds of bad behavior, but cats are more like humans," Chassman told us. "They won't put up with certain things. They don't like it when you're anxious or upset or acting out—and that makes them useful mirrors for human interaction."

Chassman stumbled into working with her rescue cat, Norman, in therapy twenty-five years ago, when she noticed the effect he had on patients in her waiting room—and has been working with them in therapy ever since. "Addicts often present a tough exterior, but when they're holding a purring cat they sort of just melt," she says. "That's important, because addiction is intimately tied to iden- tity. Part of the challenge of getting sober is giving up the identity you've created as an addict. When an addict opens up with a cat in therapy, it gives them practice at trying on a more sensitive, empa- thetic, healthier identity. Over time, they see they don't have to be tough—and that change is possible."

Indeed, researchers at Washington State University conducted a study in which they allowed adolescent boys in a substance abuse treatment center to play with shelter dogs for an hour every week; the kids ran around with the dogs, played fetch, petted them, and brushed them. After eight weeks, the boys who'd played with dogs had significantly less hostility and sadness than a similar group who had played video games or basketball.

Having a pet at home can be helpful, too. Because animals need to be fed and cared for, they impose stability and structure on addicts' chaotic lifestyles, says Chassman, and create a sense of accountability for those who've had difficulty meeting obligations. As important, being responsible for another living being provides a sense of purpose and meaning that's often missing from addicts' lives, and feeling useful can bolster people's self-worth. Animals can remind people struggling with addiction of who they are beyond their illness—parents, partners, friends, musicians, dancers, doctors, accountants—and in that way, gently nudge troubled souls toward embracing healthier habits and cleaning up their lives.

Pets Give Us a Reason to Recover

Kendyl Mason, twenty-one, was majoring in premed at the University of Southern California and pushing herself to excel when she heard about classmates using cocaine and Adderall, a stimulant prescribed for attention deficit hyperactivity disorder, so they could stay up and study longer—so she started doing it, too. "It wasn't long before I wasn't just using the drugs to stay awake and study, I was using them because I was addicted," she says.

As part of pursuing her degree, Kendyl decided to volunteer at Kitty Bungalow-Charm School for Wayward Cats in Los Angeles, a feral cat rescue and socialization facility, where a team of volunteers feeds, interacts with, and pets the undomesticated cats until they're well socialized and can be adopted. "Most of the cats are terrified when they come in, so we start by just feeding them and helping them associate us with regular meals," says Kendyl. "From there we begin petting them and playing with them. It's amazing to see their transformations. I've seen cats that scratch and bite anyone who comes near them turn into total snuggle bunnies within a month or two. It's very rewarding work."

Kendyl loved being around the cats so much that when her addiction worsened, she moved into a spare room in the Kitty Bungalow. "Being with the cats felt safer than being around people," she says.

One of the cats, Heredity, had been at the Bungalow for months. A three-year-old Siamese, she had been rescued with her five kittens, but no one was stepping up to adopt her. "She was a sweet mama. Once her kittens were adopted she started mothering the newcomers," says Kendyl. When Kendyl moved into the Bungalow, Heredity began wandering into her room and making herself at home. "She pretty much adopted me, and I fell in love with her—so we made it official and she became my cat," says Kendyl. "It was a lonely time, and I was isolating myself. But Heredity is a very vocal, interactive cat. Being able to come home and be with her was the best part of my day."

Even so, Kendyl knew her life was unraveling. "I was in terrible emotional pain, I felt physically sick all the time, I wasn't sleeping or eating enough," she says. "I couldn't prioritize my own health, but I was concerned about Heredity's well-being. So I told myself I needed to get sober for her."

In 2017, Kendyl took a leave of absence from college and went to rehab. "It was hard leaving Heredity to go to treatment, and some days I just cried, I was so worried about her—but I knew she was in good hands at the Bungalow. Now I'm in a sober-living house, so I still can't have her with me full-time, but my boyfriend brings her for regular visits. Seeing her is always my favorite part of the week. And it reminds me why I need to stay sober. I'm motivated to work my program so I can eventually be reunited with Heredity."

The people we talked to all said versions of the same thing. Sarah acknowledges that Domino provided her with the motivation to stay sober. "He gave me a sense of responsibility and showed me that I was more than just my addiction," she says. "Once I realized I could have a life without drugs, there was no turning back."

And Prince did the same for Gemma. Sadly, several years after she and Darren got married, Prince was diagnosed with cancer of the spleen. She and Darren paid for surgery, hoping to buy their sweet boy some time. It gave him three more weeks. "I was hoping for months, but it was absolutely worth it," Gemma says. When the time came to put him down, Gemma and Darren took him back to the vet and held him and petted him while he passed. "It was worse than anything I've ever experienced. Prince was my reason for living. How can you say goodbye to someone who has saved your life and given you more love than you could ever wish for? I loved Prince in spite of his problems, and my strong, willful boy loved me, too. I'd look in his eyes and see nothing but adoration. Not judgment. Not reproach. He showed me that even though I was flawed I could still be worthy of love."

For an addict—or anyone who is struggling to feel good about themselves—that kind of insight can be powerful enough to wrest a teetering soul back from the brink. Gemma's story and others like hers are moving not only because of what *did* happen but because of what *didn't*. Prince helped change the catastrophic course of Gemma's life, transforming the phrase "Who saves who?" into more than just a bumper-sticker platitude. Animals can rescue us in ways small and large—but in certain cases they actually catch us in the middle of a free fall, when the only direction we're headed is down—and through the simple force of their love, they scoop us up, turn us around, and set us back down safely on solid ground.

SECTION III

MIND

9

Cultivating Grit

Pets as a Source of Strength and Resilience

For sixteen years, Joe McCarty was a fireman and emergency medical technician (EMT) with several firehouses and hospitals near his home in Clifton Heights, Pennsylvania. He loved his job and excelled at it. In 2004, he was one of three firefighters to arrive at an elderly woman's home where smoke billowed from the windows. Inside, the unconscious eighty-year-old lay somewhere near the back door, police told them. The truck carrying the firefighters' equipment, including their oxygen masks, hadn't yet arrived, but every second the woman remained in the house diminished her chances of survival. So Joe went in without an air pack. He exited the house twice, retching from the thick, gray smoke. But on his third attempt, crawling through the scorched air, he found the woman crumpled behind the door and carried her outside, where an ambulance was waiting. Lungs searing, Joe had to spend the night in the emergency room being treated for smoke inhalation. Joe's courage made it possible for the woman to receive immediate medical care for her injuries—her only shot at pulling through the ordeal—but her burns were too extensive, and she succumbed two weeks later.

For his heroism, Joe was honored with the Delaware County

Award for Valor. And that was just one of dozens of hazardous situations he braved over the years. But the call he believes derailed his life seemed innocuous at first. He and a fellow EMT responded to a dispatch about an unconscious man in a garage. Nothing about the scene looked awry. But when they approached the garage they were hit with a noxious odor. "I couldn't identify it, but it was very, very off—and it was coming from the victim," says Joe. He and his partner performed CPR for ten minutes, and when the ambulance arrived, Joe drove the unresponsive man to the nearest ER, while the paramedics, wearing gas masks, continued to try to revive him. By the time they reached the hospital, the victim was pronounced dead—and Joe could barely breathe. "They actually shut down the ER because the smell was so bad," he says. "I heard later the guy drank a combination of gasoline, paint thinner, bed bug killer, weed killer—basically everything toxic he could find."

Joe recovered and went on with his life. But two years later, he had a stroke. Then another. And another. And *another*. There's no way to know for certain, but he believes the toxic exposure affected his brain and eventually caused the strokes. By the fourth, the whole left side of his body was paralyzed. The doctor, after seeing an MRI image of his brain, said he was amazed Joe could still walk or talk at all. "The strokes should have killed me," Joe says. In the bleak years after, he often wished they had.

By 2010, the strapping thirty-eight-year-old who had rushed into a smoke-filled building without an oxygen mask to save a stranger was unable to tie his own shoes or button his own shirt. He was prone to drooling, since he couldn't feel the left side of his face. He could barely water the lawn, much less battle five-alarm blazes. Worse, the strokes left him with debilitating migraines and seizures that struck randomly. He wound up in the ER more times than he can count. Before his health deteriorated, Joe was known for throwing spur-of-the-moment parties or jumping in the car for spontaneous road trips; afterward, he spent day after day in bed, unshowered, weepy, and dangerously depressed.

"It's heartbreaking to see someone you love so diminished," says Kim, his wife of sixteen years. "Joe lived to help people. Fighting fires was his thing. When he couldn't do it anymore, he was just completely lost." Lost in a broken body. Lost in a ruined life. Lost in a mind consumed by dark thoughts of self-destruction. "I checked myself into the hospital twice so I wouldn't go through with my plans," he says. "Every single day was a struggle, and I couldn't see how it was ever going to get better."

One of Joe's only remaining sources of happiness was Lucky, his twelve-year-old Dalmatian, who had been the fire department mascot. But Lucky was battling an untreatable form of stomach cancer, and it was clear he wouldn't live much longer. The dog was Joe's pride and joy. Kim was afraid Joe would not survive his loss. Desperate, she suggested they get another pup. A friend had recently adopted a wonderful dog through Puppy Rescue Mission (PRM), a nonprofit that partners with American soldiers overseas to transport stray animals to the United States from war zones. Adopting a "survivor" appealed to Joe, too.

On PRM's website, they clicked on a photo of a puppy in Afghanistan. The eight-week-old Afghan shepherd with a curlicue tail had been found huddled under an abandoned trailer with his siblings and mother in Wardak Province, a combat zone. Even in peaceful times, Afghanistan is a dangerous place to be a dog. Canines are shunned as dirty and dangerous, and children are taught to throw stones at them. If freezing winters, disease, staged dogfights, or speeding cars don't get them, mass round-ups and lethal poisonings probably will. Joe and Kim already knew what happened to animals in Afghanistan. They knew the puppy in the picture would surely have perished if a soldier, affectionately known as Dr. Dolittle because he has rescued so many animals while on deployment, had not found him and his family and brought them to the U.S. base. Gazing at the little dog's image, they felt heartsick. How could anyone ever harm such an innocent creature? In the photo, a bright-eyed, sweet-faced brown-and-white fluffball was lying on a Persian rug, a stuffed lion clutched between his paws. His name was Meatball. "I'm Italian and Joe is Irish," says Kim. "We knew he was meant to be ours."

A month later, in August 2012, the McCartys drove to the airport in Newark, New Jersey, to pick up their new family member. As the plane carrying Meatball and a number of other rescue animals taxied to a stop in front of them, they could hear a cacophony of barking. The dogs' handler opened the cargo hold and gave Joe the scissors to snip the zip tie on Meatball's crate. After the twenty-one-hour journey, Meatball, now five months old, took one step outside and peed all over Joe's leg. Joe burst into his first genuine laugh in months. For Kim, the sound was such a welcome relief, tears welled up in her eyes.

In the car, Joe sat in the back seat with Meatball on his lap. The fifty-five-pound puppy didn't move the entire two-hour drive home. "I don't know how it happened, but Meatball knew from the start that he was Joe's dog," recalls Kim. "I looked in the rearview mirror at one point and realized Joe's whole demeanor had changed. He looked relaxed. He was snuggling with Meatball and *smiling*. Their bond was instant, and incredible."

It was also providential.

That November, Kim was awakened by Meatball's panicky barking. She descended the stairs to the basement, where Joe slept—a habit left over from his days as a firefighter, when he'd leave the house at all hours—and found him lying on the floor in the middle of a violent seizure. Meatball, sitting on top of him, was alternately barking and frantically licking Joe's face, as if trying to rouse him out of it. Kim called 911, and the paramedics rushed Joe to the ER. But the McCartys' puppy was the true hero. "Meatball knew I needed help, and he alerted Kim. He saved me, plain and simple," says Joe. Kim agrees. "It wasn't Meatball's usual bark. It was a 'you-need-to-help-Daddy' bark." And their new dog was only getting started.

Even before the seizure, the McCartys were blown away by Meatball's calm demeanor and uncanny ability to sense what Joe was feeling. "If I had a headache coming on or felt tired, I could feel his big, soulful eyes tracking me, like he somehow knew—I mean really *knew*—I was feeling off," says Joe. Afterward, they realized their pup was an ideal candidate for service-dog training, but Joe couldn't bear to part with him for the six months of official classes, so he picked up some tips from a local training course and taught Meatball himself. "I could never get Joe to exercise, but Meatball motivated him," says Kim.

The two of them began going out for walks every day. They'd proceed down the sidewalk, Meatball struggling to rein himself in to match Joe's cautious pace, like partners learning the precise steps of some ancient ritualistic dance. Meatball would be staring up attentively at Joe, smart and eager to please, trying, with mixed success, to ignore the darting squirrels and birds. And Joe would be quietly talking to him, encouraging him, telling him over and over, "Good boy, good dog, good Meatball." Little by little, Meatball learned left from right and stop from go. He began behaving less like a distractible youngster and more like a seamless appendage of Joe—and the hobbled man by his side began seeming less like a stroke victim and more like the confident firefighter Kim had married.

Since his last stroke, Joe had become increasingly sedentary because if he fell when he was home alone, he often couldn't get up; he'd rather spend his time on the sofa, he told Kim bitterly, than flail on the floor like a wounded animal. But after Meatball mastered the method for helping Joe up—planting himself solidly to allow Joe to grab his harness and regain his footing—he began helping out around the house and yard like he used to. Ever since he fell ill, Joe had also flatly refused to go anywhere that might be crowded, because he was anxious someone would bump his numb side and knock him over—a humiliation he couldn't bear. Once Meatball learned to stay on his left flank, a solid bulwark between his disability and the teeming world, the former extrovert was willing to venture out. He and Kim began going out to dinner again, and out shopping—the small, shared activities they'd long ago left behind.

While Joe trained Meatball, Meatball was studying Joe, becoming attuned to every minute change in his posture, expression, movement, and mood. In his nonverbal way, Meatball got to know Joe more intimately than any human ever could, which helped him grasp the *subtleties* of Joe's condition—and he took his new service-dog responsibilities as seriously as any fresh-from-boot-camp Marine. When Joe stood up from the sofa too quickly and wobbled unsteadily, the dog rushed across the room and pressed his whole body gently against Joe's leg, propping him up. When he was in the vise grip of a migraine, Meatball curled up with him on the sofa, all 135 pounds of warm fur snuggled up reassuringly against Joe's back. "One time, Meatball was in the backyard and saw Joe fall inside," recalls Kim. "He began throwing himself over and over against the sliding glass door trying to get in. I think he would have broken the glass if I hadn't run into the room and let him in." When he finally raced to Joe's side, Joe just lay there and held him for a moment, murmuring, "Thanks, buddy. You're such a good boy. You love your daddy, don't you?"

Meatball didn't care that Joe could no longer fight fires. He didn't see Joe's limp or permanently curled left hand. The person he knew and loved was whole. The effect on Joe was transfiguring.

As he gained strength, Joe began taking Meatball to the firehouse to show him off. Then, when a colleague asked him to teach a fire safety class, he said yes. Not long after, he started teaching CPR, too. "I still feel insecure and self-conscious about my physical problems and the way I sound when I talk. But now I have enough confidence to stand up and speak in front of a classroom of students. Meatball did that. He gave me the will to push myself and confront my fears," Joe declares, voice quavering with emotion. "His face is the first thing I see in the morning, and it never fails to make me happy. His tail starts going a million miles an hour the second he knows I'm awake. He's always there, watching me, helping me, making sure I'm okay, begging me for treats. Since I got sick, many of my friends have fallen by the wayside, but this beautiful dog loves me, and that has to mean something. That has to mean I'm worth something after all."

The Extraordinary Trait Animals Can Inspire

Before the strokes upended his world, Joe had been a man with grit. His indomitable spirit was on display every time he strode into a burning building or approached the scene of an accident, moving *toward* danger, even as every cell in his brain screamed at him to head the opposite direction. When his health problems destroyed his ability to trust his body, he could no longer summon that extraordinary drive. But through his interactions with Meatball, his sense of determination began to grow, and that was the secret weapon he needed to come to grips with his dramatically altered life.

Although many of us live our whole lives without fully testing our mettle, research shows that grit is a cardinal trait of people who achieve exceptional success in their chosen field, regardless of what it is. Throughout the book, we've shared stories that reveal how animals can give people the resilience to pull through and bounce back from physical and emotional hardship. Think of grit as resilience on steroids—hardiness buttressed with a whopping dose of courage and endurance. It's not just the ability to push yourself hard; it's the ability to push beyond the limits of what you thought you were capable of—and to keep doing it, for months or years, or, in some cases, a lifetime. It's what keeps us going when it's easier to give up.

Angela Duckworth, PhD, a psychologist at the University of Pennsylvania who has conducted a number of groundbreaking studies that offer insight into the remarkable attribute, describes it like this: "To be gritty is to keep putting one foot in front of the other. To be gritty is to hold fast to an interesting and purposeful goal. To be gritty is to invest, day after week after year, in challenging practice. To be gritty is to fall down seven times, and rise eight."

A decade ago, Duckworth, who won a 2013 "genius grant" from the MacArthur Foundation to continue her work on grit, revealed the vital role tenacity and strength of character play when humans are pushed to the edge of their endurance. She and her colleagues followed 1,218 freshman cadets at the United States Military Academy at West Point, who were going through the rigorous summer training program known as Beast Barracks—a brutal regimen deliberately designed to test the limits of cadets' physical, emotional, and mental capacities. They measured a variety of traits, including grit, which they gauged with the twelve-item Grit Scale; the assessment has participants rank statements like "I have overcome setbacks to conquer an important challenge" and "I have achieved a goal that took years of work" on a range from "very much like me" to "not like me at all."

What they found: Grit was the most powerful predictor of who would complete the program. It was more important to success than cadets' physical aptitude, leadership potential, SAT score, or self-control. It was *the* make-or-break trait. Duckworth's other studies have found that grit is vital to everything from academic achievement to winning the national spelling bee. In other words, it can be a game-changer for success, regardless of the context. But for anyone facing long-term devastation, where improvement is incremental, setbacks are common, and hope for true change is minimal, a determined outlook can mean the difference between giving up or forging ahead and finding meaning amidst the hardship. And, as Joe's story reveals, adopting an animal can reignite this quality, setting beleaguered humans on the road to recovery.

The Battered Pit Bull Who Restored One Man's Strength

At thirty-four, Patrick Donovan was at the top of his game. A weight-training coach and competitive athlete, he had a career he was passionate about, athletic accomplishments he was proud of, and a girlfriend, Alexia, he adored. Then, in August 2014, he started feeling dizzy and light-headed in the middle of a CrossFit competition. As he continued lifting, his vision began to get wonky, like he couldn't see straight, and his left arm felt disconnected from his body and had taken on a life of its own. "It was just reaching out and touching people, so I had to hold it to my side to control it," Patrick recalls. He managed through sheer force of will to push himself through the contest. The moment it was over, he collapsed.

At the hospital, the doctors determined that he had a dissection of his carotid artery on the right side of his neck. As it bled, the blood began to clot, and during the competition, the clots traveled to his brain, blocking the blood supply and causing a stroke. As he lay in the hospital bed, trying to wrap his mind around the fact that his strong, athletic body had betrayed him, he had no idea how he'd find his way forward. "It's like Plan B. Start over. What do you do?" he says. By the time he was home five days later, he had to face the stark change in his life. "It was extremely difficult and depressing," he says. "I went from being totally busy and fit and active with my foot always on the gas pedal to nothing. A standstill. It was pretty brutal."

His friends checked in on Patrick, and Alexia spent every possible moment with him that she could. Still, he was alone for hours every day. "I might not have made it if it hadn't been for Grace," he says. Not long before the stroke, Patrick and Alexia had adopted an injured and abused pit bull. "She'd been left for dead in the middle of a street," says Patrick. "When we met her at Palm Beach County Animal Care and Control in West Palm Beach, Florida, she looked so bad. She had a bad limp, burns all over her face and neck, and a scar down the length of her left side. We realized no one would want to adopt her, so we did."

Grace, as they called her, lived up to her name. After Patrick's stroke, he and the injured pup recuperated and healed together. "I couldn't go outside because the sunlight made me feel dizzy and nauseated, so I was in a dark place, literally," he says. "But Grace seemed to know what I was going through. It's hard to overstate how helpful that can be. Rather than falling apart, I'd see Grace getting stronger and better, and I was like, yeah, just make the adjustments, have a plan, get better, and come back stronger than ever. I'd talk to her and tell her how I was feeling and share my hopes and plans with her. How could I be mopey and depressed when here's this girl who was found on the street, all beat up? Her positivity was contagious. As soon as I was able, I started taking her to the beach. I've had to readjust my workouts, and I train a lot less intensely than I did before, but I'm fit again and feeling strong. Alexia and I got married and had a baby, too. Thanks to Grace, I've learned it's not what happens to us, it's how we respond. She was my saving grace, for real."

How Animals Pump Up Willpower

In both Joe's and Patrick's lives, their dogs gave them the gumption not just to live but to *engage* with life again—and, in doing so, to redefine the parameters of possible. The question is, how did a homeless dog from a war zone and an abused pit bull, both of whom had endured bitter hardship themselves, restore human beings' spirits? As in every case of mutual rescue, there are multiple answers. Like most companion animals, Meatball and Grace gave their humans a solid base, emotional support, loyalty, and love, all of which fortified the men's will to survive. But there is more to it—and a study several years ago by two researchers at Icahn School of Medicine at Mount Sinai provides a glimpse of the other, less obvious traits that also serve to shore up and super-charge grit.

The participants were 750 Vietnam War veterans, mostly pilots, who had been held as prisoners of war. All the men were tortured or kept in solitary confinement—or both—for six to eight years. After interviewing them and giving them a battery of psychological tests, the researchers found that those who survived the ordeal *without* developing depression or PTSD—in other words, those who had grit in spades—shared certain psychological traits and social characteristics, all of which rescue animals can engender. Among the hardy vets' top assets were optimism, humor, social support, an ability to face their fears or leave their comfort zone, having meaning in life, and having a role model—the very virtues Meatball had infused Joe's life with, too.

For instance, Meatball was Joe's constant companion and, along with Kim, his most meaningful source of social support and his entrée back into his old world. Prior to his strokes, Joe had been a jovial guy who loved to joke around and make people laugh; afterward, Kim feared that part of his personality was gone for good. But from the moment their new puppy whizzed on Joe's leg, he injected humor back into the McCartys' lives—a turn of events that Kim says felt like the sun coming out after months of gloomy clouds. "Joe loves to laugh, and he loves to make me laugh," she says. "It feels satisfying to share that again."

Once Joe made the choice to take on Meatball's training, he had a mission—something to focus on that took his mind off his own suffering and gave him a sense of meaning and purpose. And as Meatball responded to and absorbed Joe's lessons, his success imbued Joe with a sense of competence, which, day by day, slowly restored his confidence. As the positives of their interactions accrued, Joe's mood became more buoyant. He started feeling more at ease moving beyond his comfort zone. And he accepted, and overcame, challenges he'd believed were impossible. Their relationship ignited the first flickering sparks of optimism.

Remember the last part of Duckworth's description of grit—the part about falling down seven times and rising eight? As Meatball strengthened Joe, he helped Joe become more adept at bouncing back from failures and setbacks—he literally helped Joe pick himself up when he fell—and that same type of valorous determination is a key component of most extraordinary success stories.

A recent study of elite athletes showed they encounter, on average, the same number of impediments and disappointments as other supremely talented athletes who don't achieve the same level of greatness. The difference: how they respond to adversity. While the talented but less successful athletes allow themselves to be thwarted by injuries, tough breaks, and bad luck, those same obstacles simply spur elite athletes to greater excellence.

Some people, like Joe and Patrick, have to summon that gutsy, won't-back-down attitude *hundreds* of times—and do it even though their sense of themselves as worthy human beings has been badly eroded. It's a remarkable feat of perseverance that requires a sensibility many strong, healthy people lack: self-compassion. And that's yet another reason the presence of an animal can be so powerfully helpful. Cats' and dogs' astonishing ability to accept us as we are, flaws and all, can often help people learn to accept themselves—making it possible for grit to become ingrained and grow.

Meatball wasn't a magic wand that cured Joe's suffering. He continued to have down days—and still does. But with his canine there for social support and motivation, he doesn't sink as low when he goes through rough patches, and he's able to push through them and return to healthier functioning more quickly. He has more grit. "Joe says to me all the time, 'I have to be strong for Meatball,'" says Kim. "The way he sees it, Meatball helps him, and it's his responsibility to help Meatball in return."

Heroic Animals Can Inspire Heroism in Humans

As important, both Meatball and Grace serve as role models for their humans. By behaving bravely in the face of adversity, the dogs reminded their owners that they, too, possess courage and resolve, and as they watched their former strays evolve into astonishingly capable and loyal creatures, both men were inspired to pursue and embrace the aspects of their former lives that they were still able to perform. They turned toward a challenge, rather than away from it. Although Joe, in particular, still finds aspects of his life difficult to handle—standing in front of a classroom of students is never easy for him—every time he does it, he exhibits courage and inches one step closer to becoming, in spirit, the heroic man he used to be.

Like so many stories of courageous animals, Joe and Meatball's saga made the local news—not because of Joe's heroics but because of Meatball's. Tales of valor, by humans or animals, have long captured people's imaginations, but there's something especially thrilling about the idea of a creature from another species coming to our rescue. Exactly why we respond so strongly to courageous feats by animals is a bit of a mystery. Maybe we *expect* humans to risk life and limb to save other humans; or perhaps hearing about animals who've displayed grit in an emergency triggers a sense memory of our long-ago past, when we relied on our newly domesticated dogs and cats to warn us of danger and keep us safe.

But I think it's more likely that these creatures' actions take our breath away because they're proof that goodness and virtue are real, that in spite of daily evidence to the contrary, there is an underlying moral order to the world after all. As Gwen Cooper says in *Homer's Odyssey,* a delightful book about her blind rescue cat: "When we see things like love, courage, loyalty and altruism exhibited in animals, we realize that these aren't just ideas that we made up from nothing. To see them demonstrated in animals proves they are real things— that they exist in the world independently of what humans invent."

Animals Can Be the Nexus Where Grit and Compassion Merge

Five years ago, Carol Skaziak, a strong-willed forty-eight-year-old in Huntington Valley, Pennsylvania, was working in public relations and marketing for a high-end boarding facility for pets when she came up with an idea for a calendar. On the cover, she featured a shelter dog, Winchester, who was one day away from being euthanized when he was given to a police department to be trained as a K9 explosive detection dog. "That story took my breath away. I fell in love with Winchester—and became obsessed with the idea that rescue dogs could become police dogs. I mean, how cool would it be if these 'throw-away dogs' could actually save lives?"

Carol put that question to Winchester's handler, Jason Walters, and together they launched Throw Away Dogs Project, a nonprofit that trains rescue dogs to become police dogs, then places them, free of charge, in police departments around the country. Their journey hasn't been easy. "I had no idea what I'd be up against. I'm not a dog trainer, I'm not a police officer—although my husband is—and the best K9 candidates aren't exactly poodles. Successful police dogs are high-energy and motivated. When I started talking to people about what I wanted to do, I met with a lot of very, very tough resistance."

The first four years were an intense struggle—and Carol felt like she was making only incremental progress. "We only placed about ten dogs—far fewer than I'd hoped—and I was sacrificing a lot: I left my job and spent lots of time on the road away from my husband and three kids," she says. At one point, the K9 trainer she'd hired began trying to change the program, and she eventually had to tell him the collaboration wasn't going to work out. "He looked me in the eye and said, 'You'll never be anything without my help.'" Then, in 2017, she met a K9 trainer with the same passion and vision for the program that she has. "He's great at this work," she says. "Since having him on board, we placed thirteen dogs in one year."

Carol is still facing daunting hurdles. She doesn't have the space to train as many dogs as she'd like. And she had to take a part-time waitressing job last year to make ends meet at home. "But I'm more committed than ever," she says. "When I was a kid, I remember the nuns in my Catholic school saying they had found their calling. I didn't understand what they meant back then. But I do now. From the moment I heard that first story of Winchester, I felt this gut-level pull to be a part of placing high-drive dogs, that are often hard for regular families to adopt, with police handlers. Now, our dogs are out there protecting people and saving lives. One shelter dog, Laika, a Malinois, does bomb sweeps of the New York City monuments, like the Statue of Liberty and the 9/11 Memorial. And Sting, a German shepherd who had problems with aggression before we rehabbed him, uncovered a biker gang's cache of explosives. I've started getting calls from people all over the world who want us to start the Throw Away Dog Project in their area. My 'junkyard dogs,' as some people think of them, are just getting started."

Carol has done inspiring work—but she might not have accomplished what she did if she hadn't crossed paths with unwanted animals that are heroically serving their communities. How did these cast-aside creatures become the catalyst for her courageous, compassionate actions?

Paul Zak, the researcher at Claremont Graduate University whose studies on oxytocin we talked about in Chapter 2, has one possible explanation. He says the hero's journey, a classic theme of movies and literature, triggers the release of oxytocin—the "moral molecule," as he calls it—and oxytocin can prompt people to behave more generously and sympathetically. In his research, Zak found that when people view touching films, and their brains become awash in oxytocin, they're more likely to donate a portion of their meager earnings from the study to charity. In other words, tales of heroism make us feel so good that they help us shift our focus from our own needs to others'. "Stories change the way our brains function—and seeing animals as heroes can be especially powerful, because it's unexpected," Zak told us. And spending time with furry heroes, as Carol does, can motivate us to look inside ourselves and make a choice that elevates us as human beings.

The same thing happened with Joe. After Meatball saved his life, the man saw his dog as a hero. Over time, Meatball's daily presence began to nudge Joe's mind out of its rigid, fixed perspective, where he saw his limitations as insurmountable, and toward a *growth* mind-set, characterized by a simple but profoundly gritty idea: The more committed he is to moving forward, the more he transforms, and transcends, his pain.

Whatever trials we face, rescue animals, through their ability to persevere, can give us the will to push ourselves to do things we weren't sure were possible. Joe is well aware that no doctor, no medication, no surgery is going to save him. He's stuck with his physical impairments. But how much he suffers and what he does with the body and life he has left, well, that's up to him. And with Meatball as an ally, he's starting to change his own narrative.

"My health problems are always going to be challenging, but they don't get me down as much anymore," he says. "Meatball showed me how to survive. He started out as a stray dog in a war zone and became a hero. Because he did, I knew I could keep pushing myself forward, too. Meatball showed me what real strength looks like, and watching him helped me rediscover that internal source of strength in myself again, too."

IO

Supporting Mental and Emotional Well-Being

Paws Anchor Us in the Present

It was a sweltering Tuesday morning in Baghdad in June 2007, and Josh Marino was walking to lunch after checking his team's equipment in the storage area on the military base that had been his home for several months. Because the threat level was considered low that day, he was wearing his duty uniform and a patrol cap instead of the heavy body armor and helmets soldiers were required to wear when the risk of attack was elevated. Josh was on the forward operating base, near a five-foot-high divider wall, several hundred yards from the dining facility, when there was a sudden, jarring blast just outside the wall, no more than ten feet away. "I instantly felt dizzy, nauseated, angry, and confused," he recalls. "As rocks and cinders rained down on me, a second explosion sent shock waves through the air, and I realized this was an attack."

Josh had just started running toward the nearest bunker when a third explosive detonated. As the base's warning siren sounded, he slammed into the bunker wall, collapsed onto the ground, and began to shake uncontrollably. "My head was pounding, and when

I stepped out of the bunker a short time later the sun felt so bright it made me flinch," he recalls.

Friends escorted Josh to the medical clinic, where the doctor diagnosed him with a series of concussions. The blasts' shock waves were so powerful they literally jolted the gray matter inside Josh's skull, leaving him with a traumatic brain injury. After the attack, he continued to perform his duties as best he could. But from that day on, he was plagued by crippling headaches, dizziness, and fatigue—all common post-concussion symptoms—as well as terrifying nightmares, anxiety, and irritability, the hallmark signs of PTSD.

Less than a year later, Josh was back in the States in an army barracks in Fort Riley, Kansas. By then, he had in many ways become a different person. The lively guy who had been known to break into an impromptu Irish jig was now so jittery he couldn't stand to be around crowds and spent most of his free time in his room with his head in his hands, an ice pack draped over his neck to dull the migraine pain that was his constant, nagging companion. Alone with his thoughts, he became increasingly alienated. "I was experiencing extreme anxiety, I couldn't focus or remember how to do certain things, and I began to sink down very deep," he says.

Josh had always relished the camaraderie he'd shared with his fellow soldiers, but his new army mates didn't understand his injuries. Concussions and PTSD are distressingly common injuries in war zones, but the devastation they cause isn't visible to the outside world. If no one can see your suffering, it's hard for people to sympathize or even acknowledge your pain. Instead of the usual brotherly support, Josh became the butt of jokes—an easy target for people's mocking and derision.

His hopelessness descended like a black pall—and he became convinced he'd *never* feel better. "I just couldn't deal with it anymore," he says. One rainy night, he wrote a goodbye letter on his computer and left it open on his desktop, along with one of his combat knives that he intended to use to take his own life. Then he went out into the dreary night to smoke his last cigarette.

"The rain was cold on my face and quickly began to soak my shirt and pants, but I didn't mind. I sat on the stoop, lit up and took a long pull," he recalls. "I felt a sense of emptiness. I didn't feel needed or loved. I just wanted it all to be over."

In the din of the rain he almost missed the soft meow coming from the bushes to his right. He glanced in the direction of the plaintive sound and saw a tiny black-and-white kitten emerge from the undergrowth. "This kitten walked over to me, meowing the whole time, sat down next to my leg, and put a single paw on my calf," he recalls. "I took a last inhale of my cigarette and tossed it into a puddle, but as I started to stand up, the kitten reached up and dug its tiny claws into my knee, trying to pull himself onto my lap. So I sat back down and held his tiny, soaking-wet body. It felt like the kitten knew there was something I couldn't handle, and he'd come over to see if he could help. It was the first gesture of kindness I'd experienced in a long time. As he curled up and started to purr I began to cry—something I didn't think I was capable of doing anymore. I thought of my mom and dad, my friends back home, and all the events that had led up to this moment. When the Charge of Quarters personnel walked by on security checks a short while later, tears were streaming down my cheeks, but a genuine smile—the first in months—spread across my face."

That small moment of connection with the stray kitten—insignificant in most people's lives—was defining. "From then on, I stopped dwelling exclusively on my problems and started worrying about the kitten's well-being and what I could do to help him," says Josh. "Every day, I went outside with a pack of tuna, and after the kitten ate, he'd hop into my lap. After a while, the black-and-white kitten recognized my voice when I called him—and our visits gave me something to look forward to. He didn't see anything wrong with me. He didn't see my flaws or imperfections. My relationship with him felt safe and made me realize that I could actually care for somebody else—and that helped me see that other people might actually be able to care for me, too."

One day, the kitten didn't come when Josh called him. Devastated, Josh asked around the base trying to find the diminutive creature. He wasn't able to get any answers, but the kitten had already given him enough hope to move forward—and one day not long after, Josh reached out to Becky, a girl he knew from high school. They began talking, then started dating. Within a year they were engaged.

Josh had grown up with animals and had a number of beloved cats as a child. Becky, as luck would have it, adored cats, too—so it was somewhat inevitable that when she visited from Pittsburgh one weekend, the two wound up at Fort Riley Stray Animal Shelter's adopt-a-thon. As they strolled slowly past a row of kennels, a black paw reached through the metal bars of one of the enclosures and swatted Josh's left arm. He stopped and peered inside. And there was the black-and-white kitten—larger, but unmistakably the same one—who had curled up in Josh's lap during his darkest moment and prevented him from going through with his tragic plan. It was a surreal moment, being reunited with the kitten, but at the same time it felt almost fated. "Of course we had to be together," says Josh. He signed the adoption papers and named the tuxedo kitten Scout.

"A year later, Becky and I got married, and Scout and I moved in with her and her three cats," he says. "It wasn't always easy. Even surrounded by all that love, my illness didn't just magically go away. Becky had to deal with all my challenges, including my nightmares that often startled her awake at night. But she and our tribe of cats made me want to better myself. I started getting out on my bike more and eating healthier—and I quit smoking. With a support network at home—one that included an excitable tuxedo cat who stuck to me like glue—I felt more confident and capable. For the first time in years, life was good."

Now Josh has a steady job. "It's a life I thought I'd never be able to have. And it's all thanks to Scout. That little kitten helped me realize I wasn't just a sack of damaged goods. Even before he really knew me, when he walked out of those bushes and curled up in my lap, he saved my life."

The Disturbing Rise of Mental Illness

In September 2016, we held a Mutual Rescue film festival to introduce our first batch of films, and *Josh & Scout* was among them. It brought down the house. But the reaction when Josh and Becky got on stage to talk about their experience was equally moving. It was their sixth wedding anniversary, they told the rapt audience, *and* they were expecting a baby. After seeing what he'd been through, and hearing the joyful update of his story, the audience broke out into a crazy mix of cheers and tears. Our most recent count shows that *Josh & Scout* has been viewed more than 20 million times worldwide—and the comments reveal the deep emotions it stirs. A man in Brazil wrote: "I confess this is the most emotional story I've ever seen." And another man's comment made me laugh. He said: "I usually don't cry at things like these since I tend to be an emotional brick. Damn it, Scout…" One woman said: "I wish more people knew how animals help people. They need to have pets in hospitals, nursing homes, schools, etc. One kitten helped one soldier. Imagine how having a staff of pets in various places would help more people! Thank you for your service, putting your life at risk to keep all safe."

That last comment moved me deeply. Josh's ordeal is so heart-rending partly because it offers a glimpse into a problem that afflicts thousands of men and women who have served in the military on behalf of our country. According to the U.S. Department of Veterans Affairs, an estimated 30 percent of Vietnam vets have had PTSD at some point, as well as about 12 percent of Gulf War veterans and up to 20 percent of those who have served in Iraq.

While combat is a high-profile cause of the disorder, it's not the only one. Because PTSD typically develops after a person experiences a terrifying incident involving physical harm or the threat of physical harm, common triggers include sexual assault, emotional or physical abuse, natural disasters, car accidents, and crime (whether you're the victim or you witness one). As many as 8 million adults in the United States suffer from the disorder every year, a staggering number for such a serious, difficult-to-treat mental illness. More worrisome, PTSD is just one of a handful of emotional problems that are afflicting greater numbers of people in the United States.

National statistics paint an increasingly troubling picture. Anxiety disorders affect 40 million adults, while 16 million adults have had at least one major depressive episode in the past year—and 3.3 million have depression that lasts at least two years. Likewise, the 2017 World Happiness Report found that, although income has increased about threefold in the United States since 1960, levels of happiness have been falling, driven largely by notable declines in both social support and a sense of freedom, as well as greater perceived corruption. In addition, the authors looked at data from three Western societies—Australia, Britain, and the United States—and found that mental illness takes a greater toll on happiness, and contributes more to overall misery, than factors like income, employment, or physical illness.

Emotional suffering doesn't just diminish people's happiness; it often creates a sense of hopelessness that can, as happened with Josh, back them into a desolate corner where it feels like the only way out is to end it all. Sadly, that disturbing notion is reflected in the latest bleak statistics as well. According to the National Center for Health Statistics, the overall suicide rate rose by 24 percent from 1999 to 2014, the most recent year for which statistics are available, surging to the highest level in nearly thirty years.

Despite the fact that the majority of Americans have more food than they could ever eat, comfortable homes, cars, vacations, and gadgets galore, many of us are deeply, even dangerously, troubled. The question of why has lots of answers. But according to a growing number of experts, our relentless pursuit of happiness is part of the problem. Study after study has revealed that none of the stuff many of us think will lift our spirits—new cars, new homes, moving to a beach community, even winning the lottery—actually does the trick in the long term. The best we'll get from those exhilarating, social media–worthy moments is a temporary blip of pleasure, and by chasing those fleeting highs we run the risk of missing the opportunity for true joy, with a small *j*—the kind of quiet happiness that comes from reading a good book, sharing a quiet meal with friends, hiking in the woods—or adopting an animal.

There's no single solution to our nation's growing discontent—which means it's important to look at everything that can protect us from despair, including all the small, daily activities and habits that dovetail with our deeper values and offer a more satisfying source of joy. While cats and dogs can bring their own set of challenges and responsibilities, they can also create a genuinely rewarding sense of comfort, support, and peace that may help sustain us through times when life feels bleak.

How an Abandoned Puppy Gave One Woman the Will to Survive

When Sarah Record, now twenty-six, was just a child, her mind became bogged down in a morass of mental illness, and by the time she was twelve, she reached a crisis point and had to be hospitalized to keep her from self-harm. Her doctors and her family thought she was battling depression, but over the years it became clear that her challenges were more severe. She was eventually diagnosed with schizoaffective disorder, a chronic, difficult to treat mental health condition that combines the hallucinations and delusions of schizophrenia with the extreme ups and downs of bipolar disorder. When she was released from the hospital that first time, however, her parents just knew their smart, sensitive daughter was deeply unhappy. Searching for anything that would bring her joy, they hit upon the idea of adopting a puppy.

"My mom took me to the local animal hospital, where the doctor introduced me to a one-week-old pup that had been abandoned at birth," she recalls. "She was no bigger than a potato. Someone had dumped the litter in an alley when they were just a day or two old and left them to die. None of her siblings survived. Otis, as I ended up naming her, was so tiny I had to feed her puppy formula from a bottle every few hours for months. She slept in a box by my bed and woke me up at six every morning, but I didn't care. I loved her and worried about her constantly, but she was a fighter and determined to live. That was eye-opening to me. This tiny creature had more will to survive than I did. And her tenacity was contagious."

For several years, Sarah's illness remained depression-like, but one night she awoke with her mind racing and a strange new energy surging through her body. "I didn't sleep hardly at all for the next few months, until the doctor finally prescribed enough medication to knock me out cold," she says. Several years later, the paranoia of schizoaffective disorder kicked in. "I became hyped up and uncontrollably suspicious," she says. "Every few minutes I'd jerk my head around because I thought people were coming to get me." Through it all, Otis was there, unfazed by her odd behavior, and ready to play, or snuggle, on cue.

"Otis might not be able to talk but she communicates with no problem. When I'm sad she puts her head on my knee and lets me cry into her fur," says Sarah. Otis also senses when Sarah's mood is deteriorating and follows her around, as if keeping an eye on her. When Sarah's brain becomes overrun by paranoia, Otis's presence calms her down and provides a helpful reality check; if someone really *were* coming to get her, Otis would know. "When I hear whispering or see things that aren't there, Otis bumps me with her pretty nose and reminds me what's good about our lives," says Sarah. "Mental illness is tough, because there's a war going on inside your head. It's not you versus someone else. It's you versus yourself. But Otis is my anchor. She somehow protects me from the awfulness inside my head."

Otis is fourteen now, but Sarah says she still has more sass and spunk than most humans. "She still spins in delirious circles when I say, 'Do you want to go for a walk?' and loves to splash in the baby pool I bought her years ago. To this day, she follows me around the house, moving from room to room wherever I go. Her devotion taught me it was okay to love myself. That kind of debt can never be settled, that kindness never repaid. I can't allow myself to think about her leaving me. It makes me too sad. To help me in the future, I got a tattoo of her paw print on my arm—a little bit of Miss 'Tiss inked indelibly on my skin, to carry with me always and remind me to be brave."

How Pets Help Buoy Our Emotions

Josh's and Sarah's stories are difficult to hear, but they illustrate an important point. Even in times of extreme depression or when dealing with long-standing mental illness, pets can meet us where we are and gently lead us to safer ground—and there's accumulating evidence that such positive outcomes may be the norm.

Over the past twenty years, studies have revealed that engaging with a pet elevates mood in a broad range of people—depressed nursing home residents, children with psychiatric disorders, veterans, married couples, drug addicts, and stressed-out students. The benefits appear to start on the chemical level. Interacting with a pet increases the level of serotonin in the brain, a hormone that helps fight depression, according to preliminary research by Rebecca Johnson and her team at the University of Missouri, whose dog-walking study we explained in Chapter 5. "A lot of the emotional benefits of pet ownership come down to a neurochemical response," she says. Being with an animal releases a potent cocktail of chemicals, Johnson found, including serotonin, oxytocin, and prolactin, a pregnancy-related hormone that plays a role in regulating emotions and well-being.

Likewise, pets often seem to understand our emotions, and a fascinating study of dogs by Hungarian researchers offers a potential glimpse into why. Human brains contain a small region near the ears devoted to recognizing voices. This voice-sensitive brain region doesn't process words but rather decodes all the subtle, contextual information voices contain, including the speakers' mood and intention, be it sarcasm, humor, or affection. To determine if dogs have an analogous brain region, the researchers trained eleven dogs to wear headphones and lie motionless inside an fMRI brain scanner for nearly ten minutes—no small feat—while they played dozens of sounds of people talking, dogs whining and barking, and noises from nature. The Hungarian researchers determined that not only do dogs possess the sound-decoding cluster of neurons but that they respond to the acoustic cues of our voices to help them discern a shriek of delight from a groan of sadness. Attila Andics, PhD, is a research fellow at the Hungarian research consortium Family Dog Project and the lead author of the study. He told us, "This ability to pick up emotion in our voices may be one reason why people feel their dogs understand them—and it's not just dogs that have this ability. Vocal emotion processing is a skill that is probably shared by many mammals. For people with mental health issues, dogs can sometimes be better partners than humans, because they offer attention and support unconditionally."

Indeed, as in most other realms, the emotional support we get from our animals plays an important role for those suffering from mental illness. A number of studies have documented the closeness between people and their pets. We don't think of them as auxiliary to our lives; they're so important they often have a place in our hearts that's similar to children. By providing meaningful emotional support, pets can feel as important as our closest friends and as indispensable as our dearest flesh and blood.

In a 2016 paper, researchers from the University of Manchester offered a glimpse of how important this vital relationship can be for people struggling with long-term mental health issues. They recruited fifty-four participants, with whom they conducted face-to-face interviews. When participants were asked to draw circle diagrams to depict the roles people and pets play in their lives, the majority placed animals in the central, most valued circle of support—and during interviews, the study subjects explained the many ways that pets provided the type of secure, intimate relationships they often found difficult to establish with people. One described the importance of pets' support this way: "Interactions with my mum, dad, and friends are all by telephone rather than physical contact and that's a big difference, [my dog's] empathic physical presence."

Participants also said that they felt their pets innately understood what they were going through, whereas people couldn't comprehend the day-to-day experience of living with a mental illness. As one participant, who identified his cat as vital to his well-being, poignantly said, "I think it's hard when you haven't had mental illness to know what the actual experience is for someone...There's like a deep chasm between us. They're on one side of it and we're on the other side of it. We're sending smoke signals to try and [communicate with] each other but we don't always understand." Not surprisingly, given the communication challenges participants faced, many also said they trust their pets more than they do humans.

Animals provided a sense of purpose and helped sufferers feel less ashamed of their illnesses. The depth and breadth of pets' effects led the researchers to conclude that mental health providers should view animals as a central, rather than marginal, source of support in the management of long-term mental health problems.

Maggie E. O'Haire, PhD, associate professor of human-animal interaction at the Center for the Human-Animal Bond at Purdue University has studied veterans with PTSD and come to a similar conclusion. "When we compared veterans with service dogs—most of them were rescues—to those who were on a waitlist to receive a dog, we found that those with dogs had significantly lower PTSD symptoms as well as lower depression and anxiety," she told us. "They also scored higher on resilience, were less likely to miss work, and more able to engage more fully in life, like attend their kids' soccer games. When we asked why they felt their pets were helpful, they talked about companionship, feelings of safety, support, and love. What we learned is this: Dogs don't make PTSD go away. But they can have a meaningful effect on symptoms. Service dogs have a measurable positive effect on psychological functioning in those with PTSD."

Key Reasons Pets Bolster Emotions: They Ease Stress and Promote Mindfulness

Stress almost always exacerbates mental illness, and chronic stress can play a role in its development. Because pets help reduce stress, that's one way they can be helpful in keeping people emotionally healthier. But another underappreciated way they soothe our emotions is by keeping us anchored in the here and now. They make us more *mindful*, which not only reduces stress but also helps us navigate the challenges of our lives with more grace. When you keep your attention on what's happening in the present moment, which occurs when you're mindful, you tone down worry (which limits our capacity to think through problems), and switch on wonder— which opens our minds to curiosity, creativity, and true connection with the people (and animals) that bring meaning and pleasure to our lives.

In 2017, *Mindful* magazine conducted a reader survey on mindfulness and pets. Of the 225 who responded, 71 percent said they felt their pets were capable of being mindful—and they shared a variety of ways in which their pets promoted their own mindfulness practice. One said: "When I let my dogs out in the morning…they just sit. Looking. Observing. When the wind blows, they lean into it. They smell it and then just sit. Then begin again."

Amber Tucker, an editor at *Mindful* magazine, told us, "Some like to see this as a matter of 'learning lessons' from their animal companions. Others find that providing loving, patient care for pets' needs can build the habit of being present. The everyday experience of being with your pets, building a relationship with them, and weathering life with them on easy days and harder days will allow you to practice mindfulness with your pet." Spiritual author Eckhart Tolle would most likely agree. In his book *The Power of Now* he says, "I have lived with several Zen masters—all of them cats."

We've all read studies about the benefits of mindfulness, but what you might not know is that there is research showing that even a few minutes of practice can reduce stress and increase concentration and self-control. Done regularly, mindfulness can even change your brain, shrinking the amygdala, the fear-based fight-or-flight center, and bulking up the prefrontal cortex, the rational brain region associated with awareness, concentration, and decision-making. Although scientists have yet to look at whether those same brain changes occur when we're with animals, it's quite possible that those of us who have difficulty meditating can derive similar benefits by being fully present with our pets.

Elisabeth Paige has found that to be true. "I suffer from bipolar disorder, and in therapy they wanted me to meditate, but I found it incredibly difficult. One day my two schipperkes came up and sat with me, and I felt so much more at ease with the experience," she told us. "I've been doing what I call 'petitations' for seven years, and in all that time I've only had one bipolar episode. I take medication, but the petitations help me control my anxiety and stabilize my moods. The effect has been transformative." As a result of her experience, Elisabeth launched a Petitations website and has recordings to guide people through the approach. "For people with mental illness it's very hard to do a loving-kindness meditation, so I suggest they start with their pets. For instance, I say the classic phrases of loving-kindness about my dog, Pippi: 'May Pippi be healthy, may Pippi be at ease, may Pippi have unconditional love, may Pippi be at peace.'"

Other approaches to meditating with pets that she recommends: a gratitude meditation in which you start with feeling grateful for your pet, then move on to feeling grateful for other beings, and end with feeling grateful for yourself. Or you can simply do a petting meditation, in which you rest your mind on the feeling of stroking your pet; when your mind wanders, label your thoughts without judgment—worrying, stressing, planning—then gently return your attention to petting. "It's easy, and it can bring you closer to your pet," says Elisabeth.

A number of others have made the link between pets and mindfulness as well. I once heard Eckhart Tolle speak, and he told the rapt audience that animals are more important to our lives now than ever. "When you look into the eyes of a dog or cat you feel alert," he said. "For a moment it frees you from your mind's ramblings and you feel your own 'being-ness.' The real reason we love cats and dogs is that we love their consciousness that shines through, and when we take the time to acknowledge it, the same consciousness arises in us." For some people, Tolle added, their relationship with a pet is the only one in which they have no fear of being judged. And when you feel fully accepted for who you are in the present moment, you begin to learn to accept yourself.

That's been true for Natalia Martinez. When the thirty-six-year-old photographer first met Willow, a five-month-old shepherd mix who had been found in Lake County, California, the puppy was cowering at the back of her kennel at Humane Society of Sonoma County, so fearful of people she wouldn't come out, even for a treat. "I crawled in the kennel with her and just sat there quietly for twenty minutes, not even looking at her, letting her get used to my presence," says Nat. "I'm shy and introverted, too, and as I sat with Willow, I felt a sense of connection. When she saw that I wasn't going to hurt her, she cautiously approached me and let me put a leash on her."

As a behavior and training volunteer at the shelter, it was Nat's job to help Willow become more social so she could find a loving home. She took Willow home to foster and introduced her to her husband, Bill, and their eight-year-old black Lab, Corbin. "Willow was particularly fearful of men, so Corbin showed Willow how to play and share toys and relax at home. She started getting used to me. And with Corbin's gentle guidance, Willow gradually began to trust Bill, too—so we decided to adopt her ourselves."

Every day, Nat took Willow for a long hike in the woods to strengthen their bond and help her get more comfortable with the wider world. "I used treats to help her cope with things that scared her. Loud noise? Treat. Kid on a skateboard? Treat. Big man? Squawking bird? Car horn? Treat, treat, treat. It forced me to be a hundred percent attentive and present in the moment—and it actually felt really good. I've struggled with mild depression, and one thing that makes it worse is my tendency to worry and ruminate. My mind gets in this spin cycle and won't get out. But with Willow, I could only focus on our immediate environment, her pace, her body language, her worried eyes looking up at me, so every outing was like a walking meditation. Being present for her was helping me cope with my own shadowy corners."

Willow was smart and eager to learn. "She mastered sit, stay, wait, and down quickly, so we moved on to things like high-five and spin and kiss. Every new skill built her confidence. She wasn't just coming out of her shell, she was becoming playful and more carefree," says Nat. "One day several years after we adopted Willow, we went to visit a local trainer we'd worked with. My once-shy dog, who used to hang back, pressing herself against my leg, trotted right up to the trainer, tail wagging. I started laughing, not just because of how far Willow had come but how far *I'd* come, too. When I'd first reached out to this woman, I felt shy and intimidated. Now, I gave her a warm hug, and was filled with gratitude—for our friendship, for her help with my special-needs dog, and above all for the fact that I'd taken Willow home in the first place. If I hadn't, I'd still be stuck in my worried brain instead of enjoying the moment. I thought I was helping Willow. But with every outing, every class, every interaction with a new person, Willow was training me to be more engaged in the present and comfortable with who I am. By keeping me more anchored in the present, she set me free."

Pets' Legacy of Love Can Give Us Strength, Too

The *Mindful* magazine survey had another response that impacted me deeply. One person said, "Pets' shorter life spans remind me to savor every moment." It's true—and reading that comment made me cry. At the time, we were immersed in writing this chapter, and my fourteen-year-old cat, Langley, had just passed away. The pain I felt was deep and all-consuming. For more than twelve years, he sniffed me every morning without fail, as if trying to determine whether I was the same person he'd enjoyed receiving head scratches from the night before or some sneaky imposter. Once he'd thoroughly vetted me, he'd spin around and present me with his hind end—a sign of approval coupled with a not-so-subtle request for me to scratch his tail. Among my friends, it came to be known as the Langley "butt swing." I realized the depth of my pain was a reflection of all the affection and joy Langley and I had shared, and that helped me embrace my sadness instead of run from it. The reason it hurts, I told myself over and over, is because of the love he and I were lucky enough to share—something I wouldn't trade even if I had to go through twice the amount of suffering.

Tragically, Josh Marino, the PTSD survivor, had to make peace with loss as well. One day, when he came home, his cat, Scout, didn't meet him at the door like he usually did. After walking through the house calling for the cat, Josh finally discovered Scout curled up under a bed. Worried, he took him to the vet. "The doctor told me Scout had leukemia," recalls Josh. "They gave him a transfusion and we spoiled him for two weeks—until one night he couldn't catch his breath. We put him in the car to rush him back to the vet. I sat in the back seat holding him, telling him everything was going to be okay, but even before we were halfway there, Scout passed away in my arms.

"I don't go a single day without thinking about him. I think about all he has afforded me the chance to do. He put me on a different path and gave me the confidence to try to come back from all the adversity I was feeling. And he showed me that I could come back. That lesson has stuck with me. I still have down days, especially since he's gone. But I've learned that tough times are inevitably followed by better ones—something I wasn't able to see before. I owe it to him to remember that lesson."

Life naturally ebbs and flows. It offers up challenges and satisfaction, sorrow and delight—and not always in equal measure. One of our core assignments as humans is finding ways to cope with difficulties so we don't sink under their weight. Exercise can help. Friends can, too—as can meditation and engaging work and a sense of spirituality and seeing a counselor.

Pets belong on that list. By giving us something to love and nurture, and providing those essential qualities in return, pets can serve as a stabilizing force for those of us who choose to give them homes. Suffering is inevitable. But so are solace and sunrises and kindness and strength. Through their resilient natures, their ability to find joy in everything from smelly socks to old apple peels, and the many ways they restore our faith in ourselves, cats and dogs are ambassadors of hope, available to provide comforting reassurance in any given moment of better, brighter days ahead.

Fostering Children's Development

*Animals' Impact on Autism, Reading Skills,
and Cognitive Growth*

In July 2016, Jessica and Brent Allen, of Bradley, Illinois, had planned to take their four kids to the airport to pick up Brent's mom, who was visiting from Colorado. But when their six-year-old daughter, Jade, who has sensory processing disorder and is on the autism spectrum, woke up with a fever, Jessica decided to stay home with her. The two of them puttered around the house, then went to the doctor. When they returned home, Jessica realized they were locked out. "I asked Jade what she wanted to do," recalls Jessica. "She's a huge cat lover, so she said she wanted to go pet the kitties."

Jessica figured why not? It was hot and humid outside, and they needed something to occupy the time. But she made it clear that they weren't going to the shelter to adopt a cat. "We already had ten animals, ranging from birds to cats to dogs, and Jade's older brother is on the autism spectrum as well," she says. "Needless to say, our hands were already quite full."

At the shelter, New Beginnings for Cats, Jessica and Jade petted the kitties, moving from one room to the next. By the time they'd been there an hour or so, they'd visited every room except one, and the shelter director, Jennifer, made it clear that the last room wasn't a good option. "She told us that's where they keep the 'unadopt-able' cats—the ones that have serious health issues, like leukemia and cancer and seizures—problems most people don't want to deal with," Jessica says. "My husband wasn't home from the airport yet, so we decided to go in."

Several cats were lolling around, but Jade spotted a blanket with a lump under it. "Jennifer said, 'Oh, honey, you don't want to mess with that cat. He's really grumpy,'" says Jessica. Even so, Jade went over, lifted the blanket, and peered underneath. Staring back at her was a scrawny, dark cat with a scowl on his face. Jade didn't seem to notice his dour expression. She sat down and began petting and talking to the cat.

The feline's name was Double Trouble. He'd been in the shelter for five years. He was toothless, depressed, and had a terminal viral disease called feline infectious peritonitis. In order to keep him alive, the shelter workers had to give him fluids three or four times a week, plus regular intravenous medications to help him eat. After spending a few minutes with the cat, Jade got up and wandered away to find other felines in need of attention.

Instead of retreating under his blanket, Double Trouble followed her. "Jennifer was shocked," says Jessica. "She said, 'Oh, my gosh, that's never happened before. He doesn't greet anybody. He usually hisses when we approach him.'" But when Jade sat down, he walked up to her, crawled onto her lap, curled up, and began to purr.

"It's hard to describe that moment," says Jessica. "Jennifer was so moved by what was happening she started to cry, then I started to cry. Jade said, 'Mommy, can I take him home?' Even though I knew my husband would freak out, I eventually decided to fill out the adoption application. This cat, that we ended up naming Trubs, had picked Jade. She loved him. I couldn't say no."

Before the family took Trubs home, the shelter employees showed Jessica how to give the cat an IV and administer his medication. "I was a little nervous about it, but we already had so much chaos in our lives, what was a little more?"

As Jessica predicted, Brent wasn't thrilled with their new addition to the family. He felt certain Trubs would live up to his name: Trouble. But over the next few days the adjustment was far easier than any of them had imagined. Trubs used the litter box, curled up with Brent and Jessica while they were watching TV, and seemed happier and healthier than they'd had any reason to expect.

What's more, the effect the cat had on Jade left them stunned. "Jade had terrible problems getting to sleep at night," says Jessica. "She's sensitive to light and sound and hot and cold. At bedtime, all her senses would kick into overdrive, and it was a nightmare. She'd get overstimulated and wouldn't be able to calm down. She'd rock back and forth, cry and scream, kick her feet, flail her hands. Night after night the same scenario played out. It was awful to see her go through that and not be able to help."

The first night Trubs was in the house, Jessica began reading to Jade, but the little girl started getting stressed and overstimulated, as usual. "I was trying to calm her down, but it wasn't working," recalls Jessica. "Out of nowhere, Trubs walked into the room, jumped on her bed, walked onto her belly, and started kneading her chest. The effect on Jade was instantaneous. She smiled, settled down, and within minutes was fast asleep. It was the best feeling ever. I was so excited I called Brent in to see what had happened. After what we'd experienced all those years, it felt like a minor miracle."

The miracle has played out every night since. Before Jade's bedtime, Trubs pads into her room, jumps on her bed, and waits for her. When she crawls into bed, he lies with her until she falls asleep. Once she's fully conked out, he heads for the family room, where he climbs on the sofa to watch TV with Brent and Jessica.

Since joining the Allen family, Trubs's health has taken a remarkable turn for the better. He eats and drinks without the help of an IV or medication. In most ways, he has integrated seamlessly into their routine. The only hitch: He isn't particularly affectionate with the Allens' other three children.

"Jade is his person," says Jessica, "and their relationship has been incredibly good for her. Before we got Trubs, she was shy and didn't know how to interact with other kids, so she had a tendency to get frustrated with social interactions. Now, she's become more verbal, more confident, and more outgoing. She'll tell kids at school about her cat. She talks about him all the time. Trubs has had such a positive impact on her ability to communicate. She's grown and developed more in the time we've had Trubs than I ever would have hoped. She knows how to count and write now. She's willing to try new things. In many ways, she's a different kid. Even Brent, who really didn't want us to adopt Trubs, looks at me all the time and says, 'This was the best decision we ever made.' Our 'unadoptable' cat changed our daughter's life."

Pets Can Lure Children With Autism Out of Their Shells

Of all the areas of the human-animal bond currently being explored, among the most well researched is the benefits for children with autism—and Jade and Trubs's story highlights one of the significant findings: Pets have the uncanny ability to reach children with developmental issues and lure them out of their shells. "Problems with communication and social engagement are among the key challenges of children with autism spectrum disorder," says Maggie E. O'Haire, whose study on veterans with PTSD we talked about in Chapter 10. O'Haire has also conducted seminal research on pets' effects on children, including those with autism—and her findings are part of a growing knowledge base confirming the social benefits of pets.

In one study, she and her colleagues videotaped children with autism in a classroom and compared their behavior when they interacted with either a guinea pig or toys—both of which the researchers presumed would be fun and engaging. "When the animals were present the children smiled more, laughed more, talked more, looked at people more, and came in more frequent physical contact with those around them, like giving a high-five or allowing their knees to touch the person sitting next to them—things children with autism often shy away from," she told us. "The difference between children's behavior in the presence of toys versus guinea pigs was remarkable. When they were with the animals, they were significantly more social, and other children approached them more frequently, as well."

In an attempt to understand how pets helped kids to open up, O'Haire's research team conducted a second study in which children with autism wore wristbands that track electrical skin conductance, a measure of physiological arousal—what most of us think of as stress. "The wristbands pick up activity in the sweat glands and can detect when you're excited or stressed," she explains. Normally, children with autism have higher rates of arousal than their typically developing peers. But when the children with autism were around animals, their stress was actually lower than their classmates'. To sort out whether the low arousal indicated that the kids were calm and relaxed or merely bored, they had children describe how they were feeling by pointing to simple frowning or smiley faces. "They picked smiley faces, which told us they were likely calm and relaxed," says O'Haire. "Our findings aren't definitive, but it's possible that one of the reasons children with autism are more socially engaged in the presence of animals is because they feel less stressed."

Pets in the home may lower stress for the whole family when a child has autism, according to a 2016 study by researchers in the United Kingdom. They found that adopting a dog reduced family strife—and the stress-reducing effect was still evident two and a half years later, when the researchers touched base with participants again. In other words, pets may have positive effects on the quality of life of the family as a whole.

A Rescue Collie's Friendship Broke Through Years of Detachment

"My brother, Drew, who is eight years younger than I am, was born with Prader-Willi syndrome, a genetic condition that affects the fifteenth chromosome, causing low IQ, autistic-like obsessions, and difficulty connecting with people," says Alexis Hurley, a literary agent in New York City. "From the time he was born, I've wanted to make him happy. When we were younger, I was always buying him things or surprising him with gifts. Drew rarely responded the way I wanted him to. My mother would say to me, 'You know, Alexis, he's doing the best he can. Don't let yourself be hurt by him.' Still, it stung. I understood he was disabled, but I thought that if I loved him enough I could change him."

Try as she might, Alexis's relationship with Drew remained frustratingly rudimentary and heartbreakingly one-sided. "Drew never said he loved me, and never hugged me nor kissed me unless I asked him to," she says. "My parents and I felt that loss acutely. Even when you understand that someone you love so much has a disability, it's difficult and painful. Drew is an important member of our family—maybe *the* most important, because of his challenges. We all adored him—and wanted to feel at least some expression of his love in return."

By the time Drew was twenty-one, Alexis had pretty much accepted that her brother's interior emotional experience would forever be closed to her. Developmentally, he was more like a middle school child, or younger. But if he hadn't opened up yet, in spite of all her efforts, what could possibly reach him? Turns out, there *was* one thing.

His name was Guinness. "My mom had the idea of adopting a rescue dog for Drew, so she and I went to the ASPCA Adoption Center in New York City," recalls Alexis. "We looked at a lot of dogs, and none of them stood out or seemed quite right. But two staff members told us we should check out a dog that was quarantined with kennel cough, so we walked right into the visit room where he was housed." Inside the kennel was a big, soulful, one-year-old collie that had been found with his brother wandering the streets in lower Manhattan. "I approached his crate, he stood up on his hind legs and wrapped his front paws around me," says Alexis.

"I looked at my mom and said, 'This is our dog.' She looked back at me. 'Yup, this is the one.'"

Initially, Drew didn't see the new family member in quite that same light. "Drew is averse to *anything* new, so when we brought Guinness home, the first thing Drew offered was, 'After this, no more dogs.'"

Guinness was unfazed by Drew's aloofness. From the minute he entered their home, the collie latched on to the difficult-to-reach young adult. Guinness slept outside Drew's door, sat next to him at the dinner table, and followed him around town, so attached to the young man he didn't even need a leash to stay by his side. "He just seemed to know that Drew was his person," recalls Alexis.

The dog's instant affection and unquestioning loyalty affected Drew in a way nothing else in his life ever had—not the thousands of hours of therapy or classes designed to draw him out and help him function, or the family's abiding love and worry and efforts to reach him. One night at dinner, not long after they'd brought Guinness home, Drew put his hand on the dog's head, looked down at him, and said, "Am I your father? You're my son. I love you so much."

"The whole family collectively lowered our forks," says Alexis. "I'm sure my jaw dropped. Drew was *never* emotional, *ever*. And he'd just told this dog that he loved him. It was stunning. Those of us who loved Drew the most, who took care of him and doted on him, had been trying for years to get him to express his emotions. And here he was opening up to a rescue dog after a few weeks!"

From then on, Drew and Guinness were inseparable. Miraculously, an abandoned collie had reached a part of Drew that no one else had access to. But what that did for the whole family was no less important: Guinness revealed that Drew was capable of feeling, and expressing, love—even if he had trouble doing it with people—and for those who cared deeply for him, that breakthrough was reassuring.

Alexis was hopeful that, as Drew became more adept at showing affection to Guinness, he might eventually become more emotionally engaged with the family. His world had a new kind of love, and he blossomed in its light. Although his affection for his family didn't manifest with ear scratches, tummy rubs, and declarations of fatherly love, Drew did change. And he learned more directly about love. Watching her brother interact with the dog made Alexis realize that affection by proxy was better than none at all. And in ways, their relationship *did* deepen.

"When Drew is feeling warmly toward me, he'll put his hand on my cheek," she says. "His efforts mean more, and his inhibitions bother me less than they used to. Seeing him with Guinness helped me accept Drew's limitations. And instead of worrying about what Drew couldn't do, I began feeling grateful for everything Guinness gave him: a sense of self-importance and mastery, an entrée into the community, the opportunity to be someone's person and caretaker, a steady source of joy. When it came down to it, those are the things I'd wanted for my brother all along."

The Myriad Ways Pets Can Be Valuable Child-Rearing Allies

The American Academy of Child and Adolescent Psychiatry, the leading professional medical organization for doctors who treat children with mental, behavioral, and emotional disorders says, "Developing positive feelings about pets can contribute to a child's self-esteem and self-confidence. Positive relationships with pets can aid in the development of trusting relationships with others. A good relationship with a pet can also help in developing nonverbal communication, compassion, and empathy."

Parents of typically developing children want that for their offspring, too. A 2015 survey of parents with children younger than eighteen conducted by the Pew Research Center found that the majority feel it's extremely important that their children are honest, ethical, caring, compassionate, and hardworking.

The good news is that despite an onslaught of news reports about the dire state of young people, in some ways, children in the United States are doing better today than ever. Rates of smoking and binge drinking among teens are down substantially since 1980, according to a 2017 report by the Federal Interagency Forum on Child and Family Statistics, which also revealed that 93 percent of young adults had completed high school in 2015, nearly 10 percent higher than in 1980, and college enrollment for recent high school grads jumped from 49 to 69 percent over the same thirty-five-year period.

That said, there are worrisome signs as well. Anxiety disorders affect 32 percent of teens, and depression among kids 12 to 17 rose from 8.7 percent in 2005 to 12.7 percent in 2015. At the same time, diagnoses of autism soared from 1 in 150 children in 2000 to 1 in 59 today. And in 2016, more than 9 percent of children had been diagnosed with attention deficit hyperactivity disorder—and nearly two-thirds of those with ADHD had at least one other mental, emotional, or behavioral disorder.

But there's reason to believe that pets add a steadying, calming element to kids' lives that can help them cope with their own personal challenges as well as those they face in the outside world—whether it's grappling with grades, peer pressure, social media, or social rejection. Studies have shown that animals can ease children's anxiety, provide them with a sense of responsibility, and give them a safe outlet for sharing their fears, worries, and challenges. Pets might even bolster children's health. A number of recent studies have pointed toward the hopeful idea that youngsters raised with dogs or cats have a reduced risk of allergies, asthma, and ear and upper respiratory infections. And there's persuasive evidence that at every age, from temperamental toddlerhood to the moody, misunderstood teenage phase, pets can serve as a stabilizing influence and offer valuable lessons about responsibility, nurturing, loyalty, and love.

A variety of studies have found that animals can build and deepen a surprising array of life-enhancing emotions in children. For instance, decades ago, before human-animal research had really taken off, Gail Melson, PhD, professor emerita of developmental studies at Purdue University, began wondering how children develop a knack for nurturing. "We looked at how children respond to babies and found that by age five, they had internalized gender scripts. In other words, they saw nurturing as 'a mommy thing.' At five, boys were already turning away from opportunities to express care to babies," she told us. "We asked ourselves where boys might get an opportunity to nurture and we came up with pets. Sure enough, when we looked at kids' relationships with cats and dogs, these very strong gender differences we'd found in relation to human babies completely disappeared. Boys were just as nurturing to animals as girls—which is important, because we need our boys to stay engaged with nurturing so they become fathers who know how take care of their children."

Melson also found, in subsequent studies, that both girls and boys formed deep emotional attachments with pets and received important social support from their animals. That solid attachment is the key to many of the other positive outcomes pet ownership has on children's development, according to Megan Mueller, PhD, co-director of the Tufts Institute for Human-Animal Interaction and the Elizabeth Arnold Stevens Junior Professor of Human-Animal Interaction at Cummings School of Veterinary Medicine at Tufts University. Research indicates, for instance, that kids with pets have lower levels of depression, stress, and anxiety and the social support they get from pets is correlated with higher self-esteem.

Several years ago, Mueller combed through data from the 4-H Study of Positive Youth Development. "I found that when kids have a strong relationship with a pet they feel more connected to their peers and their families, and they're more engaged with the broader community," she told us. "Although it's difficult to establish cause and effect with this type of study, interactions with an animal may be a way to facilitate the development of emotional and social skills necessary for creating and maintaining relationships with other humans."

Pets can ease tension in families, both by their physical presence and by stepping, sometimes unwittingly, into the role of peacemaker, according to a paper by a psychologist at the University of Chicago's Center for Family Health Research. One mother quoted in the paper pointed out that the best way to break up a sibling argument was to say, "Stop fighting, you're upsetting Barkley!"—an approach that was more effective than saying, "Stop hitting your brother." In addition, pets are also often the nexus of shared affection, bringing family members together, increasing family cohesion, and promoting interaction and communication—and they can provide invaluable emotional support for families in times of crisis and adversity, support that helps them cope, recover, and become more resilient.

For teenagers in particular, having a sympathetic, nonjudgmental soul to talk to can be a game-changer—especially for children with no siblings, who, research shows, are among the most strongly connected with pets. When Amber Kassianou-Hannan, twenty-one, of South London, was violently bullied as a teen and dropped out of school for a year, her rescue cat, Grace, was the sounding board she turned to most often to work through her dark thoughts. An only child, Amber had bonded strongly with Grace when the family adopted the cat from a neighbor who was moving and planning to relinquish the feline to a shelter.

"I was seven when we adopted Grace, and she quickly became my best friend," Amber says. "But when I was bullied as a teen, the relationship became even more important. When you're depressed, you feel like you can't talk to people, but I didn't have that problem with Grace. I could vent to her and get things off my chest, and I didn't have to worry about what she'd say back. That was really good for me, because I could say things that I knew would worry my parents. But Grace would just listen and be there."

As a result, Grace was instrumental in helping Amber make the choices that ultimately moved her past the experience and helped her get well. "I have an issue with ruminating and overthinking, and I learned that saying things out loud to Grace was helpful in breaking out of that cycle. For instance, even when the bullying was at its worst, I didn't want to leave my school because it felt like I was letting the bullies have power over me. But when I said that to Grace I realized that they already had the power and control. Staying wasn't going to prove anything. She helped me do what I needed to in order to protect myself and move on."

A couple of years after the ordeal, Amber entered a new school, where she made friends and excelled academically. Now she's finishing her university degree in English literature and creative writing. "Grace passed away this past September, and it's been really difficult," she says. "But she'll always be in my heart. During the worst phase of my life she was my best friend—my only friend, really. But she got me through. It was a comfort to know that a small furry being loved me when I couldn't love myself."

Amber's experience as an only child, and the friendship she built with Grace, bring back memories of my own childhood. I have two older siblings, but they are so much older that they were already out of the house by the time I was five—so I pretty much grew up feeling like an only child. Without siblings living at home and with parents almost old enough to be my grandparents, the animals in our home were a vital, loving, and social connection for me. Nick and Chester, two of my childhood cats, served as the glue that held our small, disparate tribe of humans—my parents and me—together, and made me feel accepted, valued, and loved.

Pets Encourage Kids to Read and Enhance Cognitive Abilities, Too

When Heather VanSchaick's son, Shaun, was four, he was diagnosed with a speech delay and struggled to articulate words. As he began learning to read, his difficulty with pronunciation sometimes made him lose interest and stop reading—which, naturally, concerned his mom. Around the time Shaun started kindergarten, Heather heard about the Book Buddies program at the Animal Rescue League of

Berks County, not far from their home in Kenhorst, Pennsylvania, and thought it sounded like the perfect solution. "The Book Buddies program has kids read to shelter cats to help improve the kids' literacy," says Heather. "Shaun had been going to the shelter with my dad, a Vietnam War vet with PTSD, who volunteered there regularly, and they'd always stop and cuddle with the cats."

Heather signed up Shaun for the program and watched in wonder as her son engaged with reading in a way he'd never been able to at home. "He was so relaxed when he was able to cuddle the cats and stroke their backs," she says. "And at the shelter he read out loud, which he never did at home, and that helped him with his articulation. Reading to the cats gave him the perfect place to focus on reading skills without any self-consciousness or distractions."

Over the past few years, Shaun has spent dozens of hours reading to the cats—and it shows. "With practice, he's gotten better and better," says Heather. "The Book Buddies program gave Shaun the confidence he needed to practice regularly and improve his skills. It's been wonderful for him. He still loves it, and goes whenever he can."

With dozens of literacy programs that include animals, and more and more schools allowing reading assistance dogs in the classroom, there's overwhelming anecdotal evidence mirroring the experience Shaun had. Now, scientific evidence is building, too. A study of third-grade students who read to a trained assistance dog for ten to fifteen minutes once a week found their reading fluency improved by 12 percent—and homeschoolers in the study saw a 30 percent improvement.

Although it's still unclear exactly why animals might help, Nancy Gee, PhD, a psychology professor at the State University of New York in Fredonia and a human-animal interaction research manager for the WALTHAM® Centre for Pet Nutrition in the United Kingdom, is homing in on answers. Her studies have shown that different aspects of preschoolers' cognitive function improve in the presence of dogs—memory, ability to follow instructions and categorize and recognize objects, even the number of words children use when telling a story.

When she and her colleagues conducted a recent literature review of animal-assisted reading programs, they concluded that the beneficial effect probably stems from a number of factors: Kids feel more supported and less stressed, which lifts their mood and their motivation to read, and they develop a positive association with reading because they like being around animals. The result: Their attitude toward reading improves, they get better at reading, and they enjoy it more—an upward spiral that ends in greater literacy, which can add depth to children's lives and one day even dollars to their paychecks. "There's strong evidence these programs are effective at helping kids read," says Gee. "I don't think we can make the claim that animals make kids smarter, but they can be an incredible benefit in the classroom. As a scientist, I was skeptical about whether animals could really have positive effects. But my research has convinced me that animals can help many kids learn—especially kids who have learning challenges."

At the same time, having a pet at home might improve other cognitive skills that could bolster children's reading and overall academic performance. Although the area needs more study, it's possible, researchers say, that pets enhance children's executive functions—the ability to pay attention, exercise self-control, think before acting, resist temptation, prioritize tasks, and adapt to changing circumstances—vital mental processes that form the foundation for doing well in school, and in life.

Caring for a pet requires a child to remember to walk and feed it—a simple, daily challenge that may train their working memory, say researchers from the University of British Columbia. Likewise, taking the time to focus on a pet's needs when they'd rather be doing something else, or forcing themselves to complete unpleasant tasks, like scooping poop, calls for self-control—a skill that's been shown to be pivotal for everything from academic success to social acceptance.

Caring for an animal also provides opportunities for children to learn responsibility, and kids who think of themselves as responsible pet owners, the researchers say, might begin to see themselves as responsible people in general—and behave conscientiously in other aspects of their lives.

Challenging Pets Can Help Struggling Children Discover Self-Compassion

At Humane Society Silicon Valley, we invite middle-school students to the shelter to engage with animals. The program, called Compassion in Action, is designed to help kids develop relationship skills, patience, diligence, confidence, and self-awareness. Many of the children who participate have behavioral or emotional needs, live in one-parent or one-adult (who is not their parent) households, have been homeless at some point, or have had unstable housing that required frequent disruptive moves. A number of these young people have already begun identifying themselves as "bad kids." But as they work with animals that have challenging behaviors, like rambunctiousness, fearfulness, or shyness, which can make animals cower when approached, they begin to make a critical distinction: They see that the animals aren't innately bad—it's their *behavior* that's flawed. By recognizing and accepting animals' flaws and imperfections, they're often able to see themselves from the same forgiving perspective.

Being able to differentiate their actions from who they *really* are on the inside, as human beings, can be the starting point for self-compassion, growth, and change. At the end of the program, one child who had been belligerent and combative in school said, "It helped me put myself in other people's shoes and see if I would like to be treated the way I treated them." Another who angered easily and gave up quickly reflected, "I learned that I can help animals and my community if I really try." And a teacher commented, "All of us saw a huge change in the way the students carried themselves and how much more optimistic they seemed."

There's a common thread in all the stories of children and pets I hear at the shelter every day: Through their nonjudgmental acceptance, animals can help bring out the best in kids. Jessica Allen saw her daughter, Jade, become more confident and engaged with her peers once she had Trubs by her side. Alexis watched her brother, Drew, blossom after developing a relationship with Guinness. Amber was able to return to school after her bullying ordeal thanks to the support of her cat, Grace. And Shaun, like thousands of children around the country, developed a budding passion for reading through the simple act of reading to a shelter cat.

Raising a member of the next generation is surely one of the most important tasks any human can undertake, and knowing the value of pets in children's lives deepens my appreciation for the untapped potential of the four-legged creatures I'm surrounded by at work every day. Animals have the ability to ground children in a relationship that's good and true and solid and real. When I walk around Humane Society Silicon Valley, I see that dimension of possibility in each and every kennel. Because of their ability to develop strong connections with kids and teens, reaching even those who are developmentally or emotionally distant and inaccessible, rescue pets have the capacity to help contribute to a stronger, more resilient, more empathetic and engaged generation of young people. In a concrete, meaningful way, the homeless animals awaiting adoption across the country and around the world have the potential to make a positive, lasting impact on the future.

SECTION IV

CONNECTION

12

Enriching Relationships

Pets Bind Us Together

When Kim and Brian Rose went to their five-month ultrasound in 2015, the couple already knew they were having a baby girl. They'd named her Aria—the first word Brian uttered when they found out Kim was pregnant. As the ultrasound technician moved the wand over Kim's swollen belly, she cheerfully narrated what she was seeing: *This is her brain, this is her spine, this is her heart.* "Then she just stopped talking, set the wand down and told us the doctor would come in shortly," Kim recalls.

The doctor told them Aria had a tumor in her lungs. Many babies with similar problems do fine and simply have the mass removed within the first year. But Aria's continued to grow. Within five weeks, their doctor in Florida sent the couple to a specialist in Philadelphia, where Kim underwent two days of imaging tests. "When the results came back, they told us the tumor had gotten so large that Aria's heart was pancaked against her rib cage. She was going into heart failure and fluid was accumulating in her body," says Kim. "I felt like I'd been punched in the gut. These were the doctors who were supposed to tell us Aria was going to be fine. Instead, they were basically saying it was hopeless. There was nothing they could do."

Kim's health began to deteriorate as well. When a fetus has abnormal fluid buildup, the mother can develop maternal mirror syndrome, in which her body mimics the baby's. It wasn't long before Kim's blood pressure began rising and her kidneys and liver began to fail. "It was the worst situation imaginable," says Kim. "We were still fourteen weeks from our due date. Delivering Aria that early would save my life but it meant saying goodbye to her. We were absolutely devastated, but the doctors advised us to do an emergency C-section."

On January 2, 2016, with Brian by Kim's side in the operating room, Aria Noelle Rose was born. "We got to hold her and be with her for an hour," says Kim. "She had such strength. She fought hard for that time with us. We told her how beautiful she was and told her we loved her over and over. And then she was gone."

For both Brian and Kim, the weeks and months that followed felt like an empty, bottomless pit of grief. "One day I was making a cup of coffee and my legs just gave out and I collapsed on the floor," recalls Brian. "It was so hard to comprehend that we'd lost Aria and nothing was going to bring her back."

To cope with her grief, Kim started seeing a counselor and writing about her experience. Then she began connecting on social media with other grieving moms. "I got lots of support, and by Aria's first birthday, I was feeling a certain level of peace," she says.

Brian wasn't anywhere near that point. "I didn't have a support group, and I felt alone and unable to talk about what had happened. People were always saying, 'What does Kim need?' There was very little 'How are you?' I just wanted to be able to say Aria's name. I was using all my energy to maintain a happy façade at work. By the time I got home, I had nothing left to give."

The shift in their relationship was stark, and scary for both of them. The Roses had met nearly eleven years before, when Kim was fourteen and Brian was fifteen. The happy, easygoing bond they'd developed early on had seemed rock solid. "We'd always laughed a lot and acted goofy with each other," says Kim. "But from the day

Aria was diagnosed, I didn't hear Brian laugh. After we lost her, we sort of tiptoed around each other. Neither of us knew how to behave anymore. I thought my husband might never come back to me."

By Aria's first birthday, the couple had moved from Florida to Fate, Texas, a suburb of Dallas, and bought a home. They'd always talked about getting a dog. Now they finally could. One Friday night, Kim was scrolling through the Facebook page of Paws in the City, a local rescue organization, when she saw a picture of Lana, a German shepherd mix puppy with pointy ears. Brian had always loved German shepherds, so she showed him the picture.

The next morning, they went to meet her. "I squatted down to pet her, and she immediately rolled over for a belly rub," says Kim. "My heart melted. She was adorable and sweet and perfect." The puppy had been found wandering the streets a month before, malnourished and infested with mange, hookworm, and tapeworm. But after being treated and living with a foster family for a month, she was healthy—and ready for a family. Brian was smitten, too, but hesitant. "I'm a planner," he says. "I like to think things through." He suggested they take a walk to discuss the choice. By the time they returned, a girl was asking one of the shelter employees about the puppy. Brian overheard her and said, "Oh, she's not available. We're adopting her."

They had to wait until Monday before they could officially take Lana home, but when Brian came home from work that day, she was there. "He walked through the front door and she came flying over to him," Kim says. "He knelt down and said, 'Hi, Lana' and started petting her and playing with her. She rolled onto her back, and her tail was thumping the floor. It was this moment of pure, exuberant joy."

The couple began taking Lana for daily walks, training her to sit and stay—and spending hours oohing and ahhing over how cute she was. "For the first time in over a year, we were able to just relax together," says Kim. "Taking care of Lana gave us something positive to focus on together and bond over. Thanks to this puppy, I was watching my husband transform before my eyes."

For Brian, the relief Lana provided was even sweeter. "Lana allowed Kim and me to have fun again. She allowed us to laugh and joke around, and to live in the moment rather than avoid it. From the first day we brought her home, we felt like a family again. And the incredible thing was how emotionally connected Lana is. There was this immediate sense that she knew what was going on with us and knew what we needed. When I'm sad she comes right over and puts her head on my lap. She just seems to know.

"After losing Aria, I felt guilty about trying to have another baby, because it felt like we'd be replacing her," he adds. "Adopting Lana made me realize that's not how it works. Lana didn't take away the pain of losing Aria. But she added joy—and that joy gave me the ability to feel my love for Aria, alongside the sadness. Thanks to Lana, Aria is more 'present' in our lives than ever. I believe Aria sent Lana to us to help us cope with our sadness and heal our family."

The Underrecognized Role Pets Play in Our Relationships

When we received Brian, Kim, and Lana's story in the second call for Mutual Rescue submissions, I was instantly struck by the idea that their experience raised an aspect of rescue-pet healing that isn't widely known. Lana didn't just ease Brian and Kim's grief. She was the light in that dark time that helped them find their way back to each other. By changing the dynamic in their home and giving them a focus of shared affection, Lana helped the grieving couple reinvent their relationship in the wake of their loss, remember the way they'd been together before they'd been overwhelmed by sadness, and renew the spark of romance.

Most of us who have rescue animals see them as family members. It sounds almost trivial it's so common. But Brian and Kim's story is a great example of how adding a four-legged family member can have significant and surprising consequences for our relationships.

Inside our homes, pets quietly serve as a cohesive force, bringing family members together and often mending and strengthening our bonds with the people who are dearest to us—giving those relationships the stability they need to hold fast through the inevitable headwinds, and even gale-force calamities, of life.

In fact, research shows that from the moment you meet a potential romantic partner—and all the way through long-term unions—pets play a surprisingly pivotal role in our love lives. Animals can be the kindling that helps that first spark of attraction catch fire (one study found that men with dogs were more likely to successfully get a woman's phone number), the glue that cements our bonds with friends and family, and the lifeline that pulls our relationships through rocky times and rough patches, restoring them to stable ground.

The love-bolstering aspect of the human-animal bond has captured the interest of some of the most highly regarded relationship researchers in the country. Several years ago, anthropologist Helen Fisher, PhD, and author of *Why Him? Why Her? How to Find and Keep Lasting Love*, and her colleagues came up with a theory: Since pets are so vital to our lives, might they also wield significant influence in our choice of partners? To test that idea, they sent a survey to a random selection of people in the United States registered on the online dating site Match.com, all of whose profiles indicated they had pets. More than 1,200 people responded.

They found that pets played a strong role in initial attraction. A third of women and a quarter of men said they've been more attracted to someone because they had a pet. And other aspects of pet ownership were even more important for how participants, particularly women, judged potential partners' overall relationship-worthiness. For instance, more than two-thirds of women and more than half of men said they would judge a date on how he or she reacted to their pet. About the same percentages of each gender said they wouldn't date someone who didn't like pets—and equally high numbers said that finding out their date adopted a pet would make them more attractive and believed that their date's choice in pets said a lot about their personality.

Fisher, who is a member of Rutgers University's Center for Human Evolutionary Studies and has conducted dozens of relationship studies, from initial attraction to long-term love, explained the findings to us this way: "The brain is very well equipped to size up whether this man or that woman has potential value as a mate. A pet ups your 'mate value' because it says a lot about you—that you're responsible, you're nurturing, you have empathy, and you're willing to take care of another creature. One of our most primal needs is finding a partner who will help us care for our young. Pets are a reasonable proxy for that trait."

Once you're in a relationship, she adds, an animal can be the thread that binds the relationship together. "Pets function as extended kin, so when you come into a relationship with an animal, or you adopt an animal together, the pet can make you feel like more of a family," she says. Pets can be a source of stress, she adds, but they can also add depth and love to people's lives that strengthens and reinforces partnerships.

Romantic relationships are among the most meaningful bonds we humans form—so anything that fortifies those connections can enhance our happiness and satisfaction with our everyday lives. To explore how and why pets can help, Canadian researchers recruited 110 people who owned pets (mostly dogs or cats) and were in committed romantic relationships that had lasted anywhere from four months to thirty-two years. Each participant answered the question: What influence does sharing a pet have on your relationship? Nearly 90 percent of the factors participants mentioned were positive, according to Anika Cloutier, the study's lead author. "People said things like, 'Our pet brings us closer together,' 'Our pet is practice for starting a family,' and 'It's a way for us to spend time together,'" Cloutier told us.

Their second study looked at fifty-eight couples who had been together between five months and fifty-eight years. Half were married; the others were living together, engaged, or dating. Twenty-seven of the couples owned a pet, thirty-one didn't. Each partner completed the study separately. On a variety of measures, the couples with pets reported higher relationship quality. "People with pets said their partners were more responsive, they agreed with their partners more often, and they were more satisfied with, invested in, and committed to the relationship," says Cloutier.

In the third study they explored empathy, to see if that could be a potential source of higher relationship happiness in couples with pets. "Empathy has been linked to both pet ownership and relationship quality, so it made sense that it might be the underlying factor that bolsters relationships in pet owners," Cloutier says. "We found that the number of years one had owned a pet was linked to higher empathy, and that in turn was linked to greater commitment to the relationship, stronger 'couple identity'—a measure of how much you feel your identity overlaps with your partner's—and more willingness to engage in behaviors that would maintain the relationship, like doing things for the other person."

Cloutier adds, "I began this research when I was dating, and I realized I was paying attention to how potential partners interacted with my two rescue dogs. Now I'm in a relationship. As my partner bonds more with my dogs, I feel myself getting closer to him. We need more studies in this area, but the most important takeaway so far is that our ability to relate to others, including significant others, is usually improved with pets."

Relationships with our pets can also serve as role models for improving human relationships, says Suzanne Phillips, PsyD, a psychologist and couples therapist. For instance, we don't believe our pets are intentionally trying to hurt us when they wake us up at night or poop on the dining room rug, she says. When they misbehave, we don't hold a grudge or bring it up weeks later; we let it go. And that "presumed innocence" approach can serve us well in all our relationships. For her book *The Surprising Secrets of Highly Happy Marriages*, relationship expert Shaunti Feldhahn interviewed and surveyed 1,000 couples to identify the differences between those who were extremely happy and those who weren't. She found that even in reasonably happy relationships, hurt spouses often assumed that their partner was wounding them intentionally. But in highly happy marriages, she writes, "wounded husbands or wives routinely assumed that their mates would never inflict pain intentionally." That presumption of innocence, she adds, is the key factor that allows the couple to forgive each other and put disagreements behind them.

The Cat That Linked a Grieving Woman to Her Deceased Sister

Pets can link us to people we love in even more profound ways. Robin and Mark Myers from Chapter 3, who lost their effervescent daughter Kylie to cancer, feel their rescue cat, Liza, keeps them connected to her in spirit. Kim and Brian Rose feel similarly about their rescue dog, Lana. And I heard about a similar story from a colleague, Bridget Keenan, at Humane Society Silicon Valley.

When Bridget's sister, Mary, was dying of cancer in 2009, she and her four other siblings took turns visiting Mary thousands of miles away in Austria. Because of scheduling issues, Bridget was the last Keenan to make the trip, and to her despair, before boarding the plane, she received a call from one of her other sisters. Mary, who was only fifty, had just passed away. "It was devastating," she says. "I knew this would be our last visit, and I was so looking forward to seeing her and spending time with her. Mary was the oldest sibling, and I was seven years younger, but we were very similar—and close. We had the same sense of humor, we looked alike, our voices sounded alike, we even gesticulated the same way. I called her every other day before she passed, but it was such a shock to lose her without getting the chance to say goodbye."

Heartbroken, she was alone the week in Austria that she thought she'd be sharing with her sister. Instead, she busied herself with the terrible task of wrapping up her sister's affairs—meeting Mary's friends, getting the death certificate, and making arrangements with the crematorium. At the end of the week, she boarded a plane for home, Mary's ashes in her bag and the heavy weight of grief in her heart.

Once home, she felt lost. Six days before she'd left for Austria, Bridget's cat had died. A day later, she'd moved into a new house. So she arrived home to an unfamiliar environment and, for the first time in years, no pet for company or support. The next day, she returned to work at Humane Society Silicon Valley, where she is director of leadership giving.

Jet-lagged and bereft, she took a midday break and headed to the one place she thought might provide some solace: Sunshine's Community Cat Room, where visitors can pet, play with, and get to know felines waiting to be adopted. If ever she needed some kitty love, it was in that moment. With Mary on her mind, Bridget sat down on the sofa. "As soon as I sat down, this gray-and-white tabby with vivid green eyes hopped off his perch and came trotting over. He popped up into my lap, put his paws on my shoulders, and started nuzzling my face," she recalls. "He was such a sweet boy, I was shocked he hadn't been adopted."

Bridget's colleague had told her about a pair of bonded male cats that were ready for adoption, so she put the adorable, friendly boy down to try to find them. "He started meowing like crazy and put his paws on my thighs like he wanted to be picked up, so I lifted him into my arms. He draped his body over my left shoulder like a baby and started purring," Bridget says. "I was talking to him and saying, 'You're really sweet. What's your name?'"

Curious about this affectionate feline who seemed so insistent on getting her attention, she pulled the card with his identifying information—and saw his name: KEENAN. She thought she must have misread it at first, but when she looked again, there it was; the cat had her and her sister Mary's last name. "I went back to my desk and looked him up in our database," she says. "He was the only animal named Keenan who had ever come through the shelter. I was in shock—and had this very strong sense that Mary had sent him to me."

Bridget learned that the cat had been surrendered two weeks before, because the family's dog didn't like him and was bullying him. Prior to that, he'd been with a family for several years. By the time Bridget met Keenan, he was seven years old. "I ran into our shelter's cat photographer later that day and said, 'There's a cat in our community room that is so friendly,'" she recalls. "He looked at me sort of funny and said, 'He's not that friendly. He doesn't usually interact with people. That's why he hasn't been adopted yet.'"

For five days straight, Bridget visited Keenan during her work breaks, and without fail, the cat made a beeline for her the moment she walked into the room. "I was still so spent and sad and exhausted, I wasn't thinking I needed to have a cat right away, but I really felt like Mary was telling me I should adopt this cat. That was so Mary. She was very much the big sister who looked out for everyone else and told us what we needed to do—and she usually gave good advice. By Friday night I started worrying that someone else might adopt him, so I went to the shelter first thing on Saturday morning and made it official. I always said that if I got married I'd love to name my first child Keenan. That hasn't happened. So this outgoing cat became Keenan Keenan."

Bridget was deeply grieving, but Keenan injected a welcome dose of love and laughter into her new home. "He was always right there with me, and he was a silly guy. They say cats don't have as many muscles in their face as humans, but he had so many expressions. He could look annoyed, wonderstruck, loving, scared. I called him the cat of a thousand faces. And he was such a gentleman. He always wanted to be by my side. If I was sitting in the living room, he'd come from wherever he was in the house, and the second he saw me he'd maintain eye contact the whole time he walked toward me. His favorite thing was to give and receive love."

The joy Keenan brought to her life deepened her conviction

that meeting him was no accident. "I firmly believe that Mary connected Keenan and me. I was in a very sad place the day I met him, and when Keenan jumped in my lap and wouldn't leave me alone it almost felt like Mary was saying, 'You need a cat, and I'm going to show you the one you need.' And she was right. Keenan helped me get through my deep loss. He filled my sad, lonely home with love and helped me move on. Every time I came home he'd do what I called 'the happy dance.' He'd greet me at the door, then walk into the adjoining living room, lie on his side, and flop back and forth a number of times to show me how happy he was I was back.

"We Keenans stick together," she adds. "And we show up for one another in times of crisis. Mary knew that more than anyone. And she knew I loved animals. I was suffering after she died. The pain of her loss, and the way it happened, weighed heavily on my mind. By sending Keenan to me the day after I brought home her ashes, she showed up in the only way she could."

Animals Keep Those Living on the Fringes Emotionally Tethered

When we think of pets, most of us envision the pampered cats and dogs that live alongside us in our comfortable homes. But an estimated 10 percent of the 3.5 million homeless people in the United States have pets as well. Whether due to job loss, mental health issues, addiction, or disability, these people find themselves outside the limits of mainstream society, with no home, no income, no safety net—and no way back in. When you see them panhandling on the street or setting up camp under a bridge with an animal, it can be easy to feel sorrier for the animal than the human. Leslie Irvine, PhD, a professor of sociology at the University of Colorado at Boulder, admits she used to feel the same.

"I even tried to buy a dog from a homeless man on the street one day," she says. The man was standing near a stoplight on the median of a busy four-lane street in Boulder. He was holding a cardboard sign that read "Homeless, Hungry, Anything Helps." By his side was a mixed-breed dog. The day was hot, and Irvine tried to give him water for his dog, but he told her he already had water, and showed her a big container full, as well as a large bag of kibble. "Even so, I was sure he couldn't provide a good life for this dog," she recalls. So she offered him sixty dollars to buy the animal. The man told her to leave him alone. She persisted, telling the man that he might have chosen homelessness, but his dog had not. Then he got angry. "I take good care of my dog," he yelled. "He has a great life. He's got food. He's got water. He's had his shots. He never leaves my side."

Irvine wasn't convinced. "In my mind, a good life meant four walls, a roof, a yard," she told us. It wasn't until nearly a decade later that she realized how wrong she'd been to treat the homeless man that way—and to assume that because he didn't have a house and a mailing address, he didn't have the heart to take proper care of a pet. By then, she'd been volunteering at Humane Society of Boulder Valley for years. "I saw a number of animals that had been abandoned by people with spacious yards and lovely homes and all the resources in the world to take care of a pet," she says. And she saw their opposite—people with no resources who would do almost anything for their animals.

The man who changed her mind for good walked into the shelter one day when she was volunteering. He was looking for his dog, who had gotten scared during a recent thunderstorm and run off, Irvine recalls. The man lived in a tent in the mountains west of the city. He had no address, no phone, no car. Even so, he returned to the shelter day after day to see if anyone had turned his dog in. "The walk took several hours each way," Irvine says. "He wore out a pair of shoes walking into town, then walking around the city putting up flyers about his lost dog. He often wept when he got the news that he hadn't turned up. I was so moved by his devotion, he forced me to see homeless people with animals in a new light. I thought, 'Which animal would have a better life? The one with this man, who loves his dog so much he spends hours looking for him, or someone with money but no real connection to their animal?' The answer, in my mind, was finally clear."

Inspired in part by that experience, Irvine eventually decided to study homeless pet owners. She conducted in-depth interviews with dozens of people who live in tents, cars, or cardboard boxes—interviews that eventually went into a book, *My Dog Always Eats First*. What she learned upends most of our common misperceptions about these disenfranchised souls and their animal companions.

She discovered, for instance, that most homeless people take meticulous care of their animals. "They make sure their animals eat well, even if it means sharing their own meager food with them. They're religious about getting their animals immunized and keeping their health care up to date, because if they're arrested for camping illegally they don't want the dog to be euthanized or given away to someone else. Their pets are well behaved and enormously bonded with their owners, because they spend every hour of every day together," she says.

And what the animals do for their people may surpass even the profound effects they have on those of us who live in more comfortable circumstances. "Animals' steady presence provides a source of consistency amid an unpredictable life," says Irvine. "Caring for an animal gives structure and purpose to a homeless person's day. They see their animals as both their best friends and their children. Their animals are often their only source of comfort and companionship. They're the reason they get up in the morning, the reason they stay sober, the reason they stay out of trouble—and sometimes the reason they don't take their own lives."

At the same time, their animals give them hope for a better life. "When homeless people see their pets as friends and family, it gives them something solid to cling to. They can say to themselves, 'I don't know what the future holds, but this animal will be there for me and I'll be there for my pet.'" That thinking allows people living on the edge to feel more connected to "normal" life and the rest of humanity.

While dogs can protect people from the dangers of living on the street, pets can also create a sense of connection and camaraderie among homeless communities, says Eileen Richardson, CEO of Downtown Streets Team (DST), an organization in Silicon Valley that has transitioned more than 1,600 homeless people into lives of self-sufficiency by giving them volunteer opportunities to clean up their communities. When DST worked with homeless people in "The Jungle," one of the largest homeless encampments in the United States, Richardson saw how important the animals were to that community. "People would feed each other's pets," she says. "Every single person knew the name of every single dog. Often, that was the only thing that brought them joy. Animals play an outsized role in homeless people's lives and in their communities."

The Gregarious Cat That Fosters a Sense of Community

Animals can bring together disparate people in other types of communities, as well, giving even the busiest and most disconnected among us a shared touchstone of joy and fellowship. And there's no animal that exemplifies the spirit of "community unifier" more fully than a gregarious cat in Los Altos, California. His name is Willy. When Marcia Chmyz and her husband and three children adopted him in 2007 from Nine Lives Foundation, a feline rescue organization in Redwood City, California, they thought they were bringing home a sweet and affectionate, but unremarkable, house pet.

They quickly learned they were wrong. Yes, Willy was sweet and affectionate. But the fluffy orange-and-white tabby, whose white snout was emblazoned with a perfect heart-shaped patch of orange around his mouth—making him look like he just got into a bowl of butterscotch pudding—was as beguilingly rogueish as he appeared. Willy refused to be confined to the house, and the more time he spent outside the Chmyzes' home, the farther afield he roamed—one or two streets over at first, then a school two blocks away and another several blocks in the opposite direction.

"Our backyard has a six-foot fence, but it was easy for Willy to climb," says Marcia. "We started getting calls from all over town saying, 'Hey, we have your cat'—especially from the local schools, which he loved to visit. We have photos of Willy at faculty meetings, school assemblies, chorus practices, and book fairs. He's such a fixture at one school that he has a spot on the secretary's desk and he's appeared a number of times in the yearbook, the staff directory, and the annual graduation slide show. He also has a bad habit of getting into delivery trucks and has been known to ride around with our postman. For a while, I kept a map of the places I knew he'd been and realized he'd gone at least a mile in every direction from our house. Willy has always viewed the world as an invitation to wander."

It isn't just that Willy's body is restless, it's like his *heart* is so overflowing with love he needs to spread it around. He roams the streets, leaving splashes of unexpected magic in his wake. "Willy loves people, and has made it his mission to meet as many as he can. I got a call one time from a real estate agent's office. Another time he was in the cereal aisle at the local drugstore. And on another occasion he was down in the basement laundry room of an apartment building, where he met a woman and followed her up three flights of stairs to her apartment," says Marcia.

With some people, Willy is more than just a passing visitor. "He regularly calls on an elderly woman who lives around the block," says Marcia. "He likes to spend the evening watching TV with her and her little poodle. He lets himself in the dog door and sometimes spends the night curled up on the foot of her bed. She'll call to let me know Willy is there, so I don't worry about him. But she enjoys his company and is thrilled to have him join them."

On Willy's Facebook page—of *course* this social cat is on social media—post after post reveals the effect he has on people. "Had an unexpected friend with us on our walk this morning. Thanks, Willy Cat, for joining us!" says one. "Thanks, Willy Cat, for helping us celebrate Nick's graduation!" says another. Yet another reads:

"Willy Cat is exploring his spiritual side this morning. He attended services at the New Beginnings Community Church."

There are pictures of Willy lolling atop school desks, wandering through a Girl Scout meeting, hanging out under a porch with a neighbor's dog, and curled up on a Ping-Pong table in someone's garage. Kids, neighbors, shopkeepers, and school staffers pose alongside their favorite feline, grinning with delight, as Willy stands nonchalantly beside them with a semi-amused look on his face—happy for the attention but clearly wondering what all the fuss is about.

"I've met more than one hundred people through Willy. He's given us a much greater connection to our neighbors and community," says Marcia. "I don't understand why he is the way he is. He's just naturally drawn to new people and new experiences. Willy is an extraordinary cat. He never ceases to amaze me. He's been an incredible presence in our lives and in the lives of many people in the community."

While most cases of mutual rescue occur between one individual and a single animal, some creatures—the dogs and cats that comfort people after mass tragedies or the therapy animals that visit the sick and dying—have the ability to enact more widespread "rescues." Willy's particular talent isn't comforting so much as delighting. Encountering him—even hearing about him—fills us with wonder and presents us with the opportunity to see that, although we think of ourselves as separate beings, we're all linked together in some unfathomable, enchanting whole.

John Townsend, PhD, a psychologist and favorite nonfiction author of mine, says in his book *Loving People: How to Love and Be Loved*, "The most important things in your life reside in your heart. In fact, we are truly alive to the extent that our heart is connected in relationship." I believe that's true—and I believe that our rescue pets can not only be a satisfying source of connection but also be the catalyst that binds humans together, helping us maintain our important relationships, through good times and bad. Bridget Keenan certainly felt more alive when she realized the feline that was wooing her right after her sister Mary's death was named Keenan. "I had the comforting sense that my sister, even though she was gone, was still watching out for me," she says. Similarly, Brian Rose was able to resume his easygoing relationship with Kim after Lana helped him see that being happy and expressing love didn't diminish his profound combination of grief and love for his daughter, Aria. Quite the opposite. "The lesson we learned is that new love doesn't divide, it multiplies," says Kim. The bundles of fur we give our hearts to aren't merely objects of affection. A stray cat or homeless dog can be the radical stimulant that makes our ability to love, and be loved, grow.

13

Beyond Cats and Dogs

Appreciating the Natural World and All the Creatures in It

When Jennifer Fenton was twelve, she was at a local park with a friend. It was dusk, and the two were getting ready to head home when four high school boys walked up and began harassing them. Her friend got up and left. Jennifer didn't. "I lived in a small town and knew who they were, so it never occurred to me that they might actually be dangerous," she says. Less than sixty seconds later, when she tried to head home, too, it was too late. Over the next hour, the boys took turns sexually assaulting her. "I was a shy kid and a good student—and the shame I felt afterward was unbearable," she says. "I thought the assault was my fault, so I didn't tell a soul."

Devastated, traumatized, and filled with self-loathing, Jennifer's life quickly unraveled. She began drinking and doing drugs, skipping school, and running away from home. She thought constantly about suicide and tried several times to take her own life. Then, when she was fifteen, her father signed her up for horseback riding lessons. Seeing how much she loved it, he bought her a horse—a beautiful Thoroughbred named Cassie.

"She was the only creature I could relate to," she says. "Riding her gave me real joy, something I hadn't felt in a long time. And being with her forced me to change my behavior. Horses mirror your emotions. If you're anxious, they're anxious. So when I was with her, I had to act strong even if I didn't feel strong. By practicing being strong around Cassie, I slowly began to regain my self-esteem. Over time, those experiences added up. Being with Cassie eventually helped me get sober, get back on a healthier path, and attend college."

As she got older, Jennifer's life got busier, and she eventually sold Cassie. But in 2016, she returned to a stable and started riding again. Within weeks she was inspired to start the Equine Healing Collaborative (EHC), a therapy center that offers Mindful Equine Assisted Psychotherapy, a treatment model that combines activities with horses and elements of traditional therapy, including mindfulness. "Being around horses brought it all back to me. I remembered how healing Cassie had been for me and wanted to be able to pass that gift along to others," she says.

Today, at forty-seven, Jennifer is a marriage and family therapist in Carmel, California, and has a therapy herd of nine rescue animals, all of whom were taken from neglectful or abusive situations: two miniature horses, three donkeys, and four horses.

"When Nutter and Butter, our miniature horses, got here, they were almost feral," Jennifer says. "It took them two months to settle in, but now they're gentle and kind and do their jobs extremely well. My team and I use them in empathy courses for children in foster care, many of whom have been abused and neglected. Without secure attachment to their primary caregivers, children often don't have the opportunity to develop empathy and other essential social skills. We have the kids do a brushing activity with Nutter and Butter to help them learn how to pay attention to body language and respond appropriately. Over the course of the sessions we see the kids learning to be gentle and patient and watch the horses for cues. Nutter and Butter are able to convey far more information about appropriate behavior in one session than I could alone in twenty."

Jennifer and her team also provide mental health counseling for victims of sex trafficking. "In one session, we had a participant who had been trafficked as a child by her own mother. There's no greater form of abandonment than that," Jennifer says. "Understandably, she was very guarded emotionally. I wasn't sure we'd be able to reach her. Then Sarah, one of our donkeys, walked right up to her and nuzzled her. The woman's whole demeanor changed. She spent the full forty-minute session sobbing into Sarah's fur. My staff and I all had goose bumps. Here was this sentient being that could have walked away at any time during those forty minutes. But Sarah just stood there and allowed this woman to pour her grief out. When you hear that donkeys are beasts of burden, they really are. They're willing to carry heavy loads of emotional trauma. We didn't prompt Sarah, or train her or entice her with food. She sensed suffering and moved toward it. I can't explain how or why Sarah knew that woman needed her. But she did. That session with Sarah was the first time she'd felt safe enough to express her emotions."

The horses and donkeys have continued to heal Jennifer as well—especially Lola, a horse that someone brought to the EHC property last year, in the hope that Jennifer would adopt her, along with a pair of neglected donkeys. "When I first met Lola, what struck me most was the sheer look of despair on her face. She was clearly in pain, although at the time I didn't know what was causing it," Jennifer recalls. "I'm ashamed to say I tried to ignore her suffering at first. We didn't have the time or the money to deal with an injured horse.

"But one night I felt so sorry for her I tried to massage her—and that forced me to acknowledge her agony. I could no longer look away. I called a vet, who diagnosed her with a broken pelvis and shoulder. We adopted her, treated her, and rehabilitated her. Looking back, I see that part of my avoidance of Lola's pain had to do with my inability to acknowledge my own pain. Lola reminded me too much of myself. But confronting Lola's pain gave me the opportunity—after years of looking away—to confront my own. Not long ago, I had the strength to return to my hometown and attend an event where I came face-to-face with people who witnessed or participated in the bullying my perpetrators did to me.

I even stood up in front of everyone and spoke a little about my work. I felt strong and proud and whole. For the first time, the traumatized twelve-year-old child and the forty-seven-year-old woman were one. Like Lola's broken bones, my fractured heart has healed."

Mutual Rescue Isn't Just About Dogs and Cats

Humans can save and be saved by a variety of creatures. People form meaningful bonds with rabbits and rats, snakes and reptiles, birds and bats, sheep, pigs, goats, and chickens. And horses' ability to help suffering people find their way to a better place is so well established it's become part of a widely accepted offshoot of traditional psychotherapy. In equine-assisted psychotherapy (EAP), as it is known, people who are struggling socially or emotionally—from a child with autism to a veteran with PTSD—are guided by a therapist on a variety of simple ways to interact with a horse. You might walk the horse around a ring, say, or lead it through a series of cones, or brush and groom the animal. As you go through the exercises, emotions come up spontaneously, so you get a chance to recognize those feelings, whether it's anxiety, anger, fear, sadness, grief, or insecurity, and modify them in the moment. You learn by doing, rather than talking, which can sometimes offer more powerful and lasting lessons. Through those interactions, and the horse's response to the interactions, people often are able to gain remarkable insight into the issues that trouble them.

Scientific evidence of EAP's effectiveness is building, along with its popularity. Researchers at Florida Atlantic University in Jupiter recently tested the approach in people with PTSD and anxiety and found a 25 percent and 30 percent decrease in symptoms, respectively, after six two-hour sessions. The approach has also been shown to be effective for abused women—who, by working with horses, gain confidence and the ability to trust and create positive attachments—as well as at-risk adolescents and autistic children.

Horses are valuable collaborators in therapy partly because

they're prey animals. Naturally wary and highly attuned to their environment, particularly other living creatures, they have an almost uncanny ability to tap into, and take on, human emotions. As Jennifer pointed out, if you're anxious, they're anxious. Thanks to their keen emotional acuity, therapy horses serve as both mirror and guide, reflecting the challenging emotions clients are dealing with and, as a result, giving people the opportunity to understand their own minds and get control of them. The reward: When clients are able to settle into a composed, calm, self-confident state, the horse trusts them and responds in kind. In a concrete way, EAP gives people the chance to practice being their best selves.

Horses are an ancient species. They've survived for nearly 55 million years, another reason they're adept at assessing situations—and tremendously intuitive, says Danielle MacKinnon, an animal communicator, intuitive, and author of *Animal Lessons: Discovering Your Spiritual Connection with Animals*. In her Horse and Soul program with Eponicity in Costa Rica, the horses—most of whom are rescues—choose which participants they want to work with, rather than the other way around. "Participants sit in chairs around the ring, and the horses walk around, one by one, sensing and considering everyone before they settle on someone to work with," she says. "I'm sometimes surprised at who they pick, but by the end of the week it's always clear why they chose the person they did."

In a 2017 workshop, for instance, Charlie, a regal horse, chose Lisa (not her real name), a woman who felt let down by her social support network and as a result was isolating herself. "She was shy and held herself at a distance from the group, listening and observing but rarely speaking," says MacKinnon.

In her early sessions with Charlie, she made herself small and stood away from him. The turning point for Lisa came when the facilitators challenged her to lie on Charlie's bare back. "With Charlie standing patiently and the team members surrounding the two of them, Lisa eventually allowed herself to relax onto Charlie's back," recalls MacKinnon. "Lisa began crying as she melted into his embrace. By trusting him and allowing him to help her, she was able to truly connect with another living being for the first time in years."

The experience was so powerful she was able to carry it forward into the rest of her life. Lisa joined MacKinnon's online community and began reaching out and sharing her experience with others, and she has decided to begin the training protocol to become a practitioner of animal communication. "Charlie showed her how to live from a place of trust and love rather than fear, and it changed her life," says MacKinnon.

Incredible as they are, horses are just one of a breathtaking array of animals being used for therapeutic purposes these days. The trend to embrace diverse species reveals that even the most unusual creatures that live in our midst are relatable when we get to know them. A clinic in London has used corn snakes, nonvenomous reptiles that enjoy being touched, for instance, in their treatment programs for addiction and eating disorders. Handling them, doctors say, gives patients a sense of accomplishment and purpose. Therapists sometimes use turtles in sessions with children.

With the rise of social media and images of people with their pets, the surprising range of creatures with whom humans can forge meaningful bonds—bats, mice, hedgehogs, ferrets, and all manner of birds—has become ever more apparent. The stories that emerge from these relationships reveal that humans can connect with an array of species. When they do, they often discover a deep sense of kinship and eye-opening lessons about other beings' lives and who and what we deem lovable.

How a Rescue Pig Helped a Woman Heal—and Changed Her Life

Over Labor Day weekend in 2013, Erin Brinkley-Burgardt was rear-ended while driving. The force of the impact caused a serious concussion, and Erin, who was not only working but also going to school to get her master's degree in business, was suddenly forced to retreat from all her activities and rest. "I had motion sickness, difficulty concentrating and focusing, and short-term memory loss, so I had to drop out of my graduate school coursework," says the thirty-three-year-old, of Deer Trail, Colorado. "All I could do was lie on the couch and allow my brain to heal. I wasn't allowed to read or look at a TV or computer screen. I'm hyper-motivated and don't do well with downtime, so it was difficult for me, mentally and emotionally."

She struggled with moments of sadness and depression, but there was one thing that prevented her from sinking too low: Pippy, her potbellied pig. Erin and her husband had adopted Pippy four months before the accident, after seeing an ad for an unwanted pig online. "Pigs have been my favorite animal since I was six—probably because of *Charlotte's Web*, my favorite childhood book," she says. "Even so, we really didn't know what we were getting into when we adopted her. She was five months old and only weighed twenty pounds—but pigs are far more challenging than puppies. They're like toddlers. They're super smart, so they can figure out how to get into just about anything. We had a twenty-gallon container of dog food, and we came home from work one day and there was Pippy in the bottom of it. She'd managed to get the lid off and spent the day eating away. Another time she climbed up onto a swivel chair to get the cat food on the counter. We had to childproof the entire house to keep her safe and healthy."

Pigs are also extremely social and emotional—which proved to be game-changing after Erin's accident. "She knew I was in emotional distress, even if I wasn't crying or acting sad. She watched over me the whole time I was stuck at home. If I was on the couch, she wanted to be in my lap or snuggling alongside me. Pippy knew I was down. She knew I was struggling."

After Erin recovered, she and her husband were so enamored of Pippy they decided to rescue a second pig. "In the process of looking for another pig who had been orphaned, we realized there's a huge need for pig rescue in this country," she says. "Too many people adopt pigs without knowing what they're getting into, and breeders often don't make it clear how large the animals are going to get. Less than five percent of pigs stay with their original family their whole lives. These poor animals are constantly being abandoned. We were so concerned and upset by the problem that, after we adopted our second pig, Boris, we decided to start a pig rescue."

The couple thought it would take roughly five years to get the project up and running. Within six months the organization was going hog wild. "We launched in August 2014 and had to move to a property forty miles east of Denver very quickly to accommodate the animals. We had eight pigs at that point. Now we've moved to an even larger property in Deer Trail, where we have eighty-six pigs—although we've rescued more than a hundred fifty, all told."

In the spring of 2014, Erin, who learned while she was healing from her concussion how soothing and uplifting the presence of a pig could be, began working with Pippy and Boris as therapy pigs. First, she took them to memory care facilities for people with various types of dementia and then branched out to visits with other groups—mentally disabled people, schoolchildren, senior citizens. "So many people have an innate desire to interact with animals," she says. "In our school visits, the pigs help kids focus. With mentally disabled people, the pigs bring them incredible joy. At the memory care facility, the pigs draw people out and engage them. A lot of folks in the nursing homes here grew up on farms, so the pigs bring back memories of their childhood. We've had completely nonverbal people start to communicate after a visit from Pippy or Boris. It's been wonderfully rewarding."

Pigs, she adds, have astonishingly high emotional intelligence and perceive, and experience, deep feelings. "In 2015, we took on Chopper, a big male pig who had been surrendered in a divorce. He was five years old, and that was the only family he'd ever known. After coming to the farm, he cried for two weeks straight. There were real tears rolling down his face. Pigs always go through a period of grieving and depression after their families give them up. But this poor guy was totally heartbroken. We gave him lots of extra attention and treats to try to rebuild his trust. Pigs' emotions are very much like humans'. Their sadness can go incredibly deep.

"So can their joy," she adds. "When the pigs are excited and happy, they cruise around in circles as fast as they can. Plastic bags delight them, as does cardboard. Or stealing a bag of treats. They'll go running off with it, delirious with joy," she says. "There are times when I'm watching them that my jaw just drops. Pigs are far more amazing than most people realize. They're one of the most emotionally intelligent creatures on earth—right up there with humans. We had a handicapped visitor to the sanctuary last year. She suffers from physical and mental disabilities and is nonverbal. When we were showing her around, three of our therapy pigs—Pippy, Boris, and Pumba—surrounded her wheelchair for attention. It was a beautiful moment. These three pigs, based on their experiences as therapy pigs, knew that this visitor was different and special and came around to make sure she had a wonderful experience at the sanctuary. I can't describe how moving that was. I wish more people could understand that, despite the fact that we all come in different shapes and forms, all living creatures are far more alike than we realize."

Animals Provide Much-Needed Connection to the Natural World

Although stories like Erin's may sound surprising, they shouldn't. Our strong emotional response with a variety of animals actually seems to be innate—a relic of a long-ago time when humans saw themselves as part of the fabric of the natural world, one animal species among many, rather than separate from it. Researchers have found, for instance, that infants smile more at a live rabbit than a toy one, and babies as young as six months old try to get closer to and make more physical contact with dogs and cats than battery-powered pets—signs that we're born with a love of animals, or at least a fascination. And that attraction seems to be interwoven with our innate reverence for the wild places from which we all evolved. Indeed, a concept known as "biophilia" posits that we all have not only an instinctive urge to form close emotional bonds with non-human animals but also a built-in affinity for nature itself.

A surge in research showing the calming effects of spending time in nature offers tangential support for this idea. A fifteen-minute walk in the woods causes a dramatic drop in the stress hormone cortisol, according to Japanese researchers, along with a measurable drop in heart rate and blood pressure. When we enter a green, leafy space, our bodies relax. It's almost as if, on some deep level, we recognize we're home.

Because animals retain a congenital kinship with the outdoors, they're likely to keep us linked to the living world around us—and the desire to have a pet may stem partly from our inborn craving to have a closer relationship with untamed places, says Barbara King, an anthropologist and author of *Being with Animals: Why We Are Obsessed with the Furry, Scaly, Feathered Creatures Who Populate Our World*. "We are animals, too, after all, and we have shared so much of our evolutionary journey on Earth with other beings out in the wild, that a chance to share our emotional and physical space with pets on a daily basis can bring immense pleasure, especially in a fast-paced, hyper-technological world. With my five rescued cats, even though of course they're domesticated animals, I love to see that wildness when their true cat natures emerge in play or interaction."

My cat Langley, who passed away while we were writing this book, was a reliable ambassador for the natural world. Whenever I'd receive flowers, he'd sniff them. He'd nuzzle his face into the blossoms. He'd lie down next to them. It was as if being in their vicinity brought him some sort of special, ethereal joy—and his appreciation gave me the opportunity to pay even more attention to their remarkable beauty. His behavior encouraged me to look at flowers—*really* look—and when I did, I was inevitably stirred by the simple grace of nature.

Animals, whether we recognize it consciously or not, keep us rooted in nature—and they help us appreciate its beauty, mystery, and joy. Dogs, in particular, are likely to literally pull us outside—as if we're leashed to them, and not the other way around. Thanks to them we're often able to remove our human blinders and look up at a tree or the sky or down at a bed of forget-me-nots underfoot and see the marvel of it all through their eyes. That squirrel! That stick! That meadow! By enlarging our awareness and appreciation of the natural world, they may even bolster our sense of responsibility to protect it.

Having Animals in Our Lives May Help Us Become Better People

What's truly remarkable is that being in nature doesn't just lower our stress and affect our physiology, it often transforms us emotionally—helping us transcend our usual focus on ourselves and become more cooperative, giving, and caring. When researchers at Carleton University in Canada had study subjects watch either a video of a stunning architectural tour of New York City or a BBC documentary called *Planet Earth* with extraordinary panoramas of nature, then play a fishing-related video game in which players' choices determined the future health of the ocean, they discovered something remarkable.

"About seventy-one percent of the time the people who saw the BBC video fished sustainably, compared to fifty percent of people who watched the architecture video," John Zelenski, PhD, a professor of psychology at Carleton University, told us. "When paired with findings of other similar studies, our conclusion was this: Nature doesn't just make people healthier. It makes them *nicer*."

Although no one knows for sure what it is about being in nature that makes us more caring, one theory is that outdoor settings often inspire the reverent feeling of awe—an ennobling and surprisingly important emotion that seems to be hardwired into the human experience, according to Jennifer Stellar, PhD, assistant professor of psychology at the University of Toronto in Mississauga.

Stellar and her former colleagues at the University of California at Berkeley have conducted much of the seminal research on awe over the past decade, and they have found that the sensation is associated with inspiration, gratitude, curiosity, and a desire to explore. "Awe makes us feel both related to others and the world around us—more aware of the 'oneness' of life—and at the same time humbled and insignificant, a tiny speck of dust in the vastness of the universe," Stellar told us. "And you don't have to travel to distant places to feel it. Awe can come from an experience in your own backyard that challenges the way you see the world." No matter where you are when it comes over you, the feeling of wonder can be a way to move beyond your limited physical and mental experience and tiptoe toward a mind-set that's more inclusive and profound.

The sensation of awe is experienced similarly by different cultures around the world, research shows, so it appears to be woven into our DNA. Researchers speculate that the reason we're wired to feel awe is its ability to help us act in more collaborative ways, thereby safeguarding our survival. Studies have affirmed that by dissolving our sense of ourselves as separate individuals and positioning us within a larger context, awe can encourage us to act more generously, ethically, and fairly.

In media interviews, astronauts inevitably talk about the astonishment they experienced looking back at Earth from space—a sensation known as "the overview effect." Many muse on how they could see for the first time the fragility of our planet, and realized we all have a fundamental responsibility as Earth's inhabitants to protect it. As Scott Carpenter, one of the original seven Mercury astronauts, said in a 1992 speech: "This planet is...a delicate flower and it must be cared for. It's lonely. It's small. It's isolated, and there is no resupply. Clearly the highest loyalty we should have is not to our own country or our own religion or our hometown or even to ourselves. It should be to, number two, the family of man, and number one, the planet at large. This is our home, and this is all we've got." Awe-inspiring incidents don't just temporarily give us lift, they can fundamentally alter the way we approach the world, and in doing so, they offer us a unique gift: They shift our thinking from *me* to *we*.

And we don't need to travel to space to experience it. Even a brief, awe-inducing encounter with the majesty, mystery, or beauty of nature, studies show, can bring forth people's ability to take on the concerns of others and see themselves as part of a broader collective. And animals, from the wild ones who roam the woods to the creatures who live on farms to the cuddly pets snuggled beside you on the sofa, seem to serve as a proxy for nature at large. "Pets provide a possible link to nature—and in our studies, people who own pets score higher on questionnaires that gauge how deeply connected you feel to nature," says Zelenski.

Barbara King, also author of *Personalities on the Plate: The Lives & Minds of Animals We Eat*, agrees. "In the best of our pet-keeping urges, we accomplish an important thing: using our relationship with our pets as a window through which to empathize with other animals who also think and feel, including farmed animals," she says. "I no longer see any difference between loving the dog in our home and loving the pig or chicken we choose not to put on our plate."

A horse's ability to tap into our emotions, a crying pig, a donkey comforting a grieving woman, or a cat that adores flowers—any of a number of everyday interactions with animals can trigger the awareness that we're just one small part of a vast, enigmatic whole, a sensation that can help us feel more charitable, generous, and concerned for the well-being of others, and even the planet as a whole.

And some people who have benefited from animals are inspired to help others heal, too. When Jennifer started the Equine Healing Collaborative, she says her goal was to provide a path to self-discovery, recovery, personal growth, and reconnection to the natural world—the same things she'd found through her interactions with her first horse, Cassie. She felt so awed by what Cassie had done for her, and what she believed horses could do for others, that she has a generous sliding scale so anyone who is interested in the approach can have access to it. "Being with horses turned my life around. I know how grounding that connection with an animal can be," she says. "Now, my goal is twofold: I want to rescue as many neglected horses and donkeys as I can—and share their healing influence with as many people as possible."

Likewise, Erin's capacity for love and providing help grew exponentially after adopting her first pig, Pippy. "This life we've created by rescuing pigs is something I never would have dreamed of a decade ago, and yet I can't imagine doing anything else now," she says. "Within a very short amount of time I went from working and focusing on getting my master's degree in business and being intensely career-driven to opening a pig rescue. You don't get a much more dramatic turnaround than that. Pippy didn't just open my eyes to the hidden depths of her species. She opened my heart."

Our adopted rescue cats and dogs can enhance our ability to care for others as well. By offering us a deeply rewarding bond, and keeping us grounded in the wild world, shelter pets give us the opportunity to expand our awareness and concern for a variety of creatures that inhabit our planet. Moreover, living with animals on a daily basis, enjoying their company, and seeing the beauty of nature through their eyes can help us rise above our human differences and appreciate the value of all living beings, as well as the magnificent wild places that surround us that are no less deserving of protection. Living with animals is a reminder of the awe and wonder of life itself. Pay attention. Their meows and bow-wows might just mean "Wow."

14

Discovering Purpose

*What Animals Can Teach Us About
Meaning, Love, and Faith*

In August 2015, when LaVonne Bower, of Bradenton, Florida, agreed to foster Oz, a pit bull mix whose left rear leg had been shattered by a car, she was apprehensive about what she was getting into. For one thing, she'd been struggling with low-grade depression. In her early forties, she was happily married, had a teenage son and a good-job at an insurance company. Even so, she was tormented by the feeling that her life lacked meaning. She felt, in her words, like she was "wasting the gift of life." On top of that, Oz wasn't exactly a simple foster dog. "He was about to have surgery to amputate his injured leg, and we already had two dogs at home with health issues," she says. "I thought we might be taking on too much."

Then, she met Oz at Nate's Honor Animal Rescue in Bradenton. "He limped out of the kennel, his tail wagging, and curled up in my lap. He looked up at me with these beautiful brown eyes, and I knew he wasn't a foster dog. Oz was *our* dog," she says.

After she and her husband brought Oz home, they began to see how extraordinary their new family member really was. "When Oz was in crowds of people he was incredibly gentle and calm," she says. "One of the things I'd been dreaming about was getting a therapy dog so I could work with the elderly and ill and wounded veterans. My other two dogs were wonderful, but neither of them had the right temperament. As I watched Oz interact with strangers, I knew he was the one I'd been waiting for. He was so sweet and attentive and tender. It was like he was born to provide comfort."

Several months later, Oz passed his therapy dog certification test, and they began visiting patients at the Veterans Administration hospital near their home. "Oz seemed to know instinctively what to do. We met with hospice patients and retired veterans and cancer and recreational therapy patients, and every single person brightened when Oz walked in the room," she says. "There's something about a happy-go-lucky three-legged dog that just gives you *hope*. Veterans with injuries could especially relate to Oz because he is missing a leg. They could see that he'd been wounded, too."

LaVonne relished the effect her new dog had on patients, but the work was sporadic, and she was eager to do more. "My stepfather was a World War II veteran and my husband had been in the military. I've always had a lot of respect for people who serve," she says. "So I started putting together a nonprofit, Paws and Warriors, to help match rescue dogs with veterans who could benefit from having a loving companion at home."

In September 2016, just as she began mapping out the logistics of her new venture, she was taking off her exercise bra one day after a workout and felt a lump in her breast. "I knew it was bad the minute I felt it," she says. "I called my doctor and asked to be seen right away." An ultrasound and mammogram confirmed the diagnosis: LaVonne had breast cancer, and it had already spread to her lymph nodes. "I was scared and worried—and heartbroken to think that all the work Oz and I had done might be over," she says. "We were just getting started. Suddenly it felt like I was watching my dream disappear."

Treatment took the better part of a year. She underwent a double mastectomy, spent months recuperating, then endured four months of harsh chemotherapy, followed by two months of radiation. On the second day after her chemo treatments, the chemicals kicked in, making her sick and miserable. "All I could do was sit on the couch. I felt completely hollowed out. But Oz would crawl into my lap and curl up in a little ball," she recalls. "His missing leg was a reminder that he'd been through his own ordeal. I'd tell myself, 'If he can survive the loss of a limb, I can deal with cancer.' No matter how scared I was or how sick and tired I felt, Oz made me feel like everything was going to be all right." Her other dogs were wonderful, too. Throughout her treatment, all three canines rallied around her like sentinels, rarely leaving her side. "They had to be touching me at all times—a head in my lap, a paw on my leg, a warm body leaning against me," she says. "In their doggy way, they were doing what they could to take care of me. It was absolutely healing."

When she felt low, she cheered herself up by thinking about her nonprofit. "Planning my next steps gave me a sense of purpose and motivated me to stay strong. I truly felt like Oz and I had unfinished business, and nothing, not even cancer, was going to prevent us from making a difference."

When the final treatment was over, she resumed networking with veterans. Still bald from chemo, she reached out to shelters across the country and started matching veterans she'd met through Oz with service dogs. Within twelve months, she placed twenty-four rescue dogs with vets who suffered from PTSD or depression or were wheelchair-bound—and had numerous potential matches in the pipeline. "It's been extremely gratifying to see my vision come together and see the effect the animals have on veterans," she says. "In some cases, it has turned their lives around.

"All the good things that have happened started with Oz. I never would have had these opportunities if it weren't for the work I was doing with him. He and I even flew to New York at one point to meet new business contacts. I'm an introvert. I never would have had the courage to do that if Oz hadn't been by my side. There's a chance my cancer will come back down the road, which is a scary thing to live with. But none of us know what life has in store. Cancer helped me see that. It made me grateful to be alive. But Oz helped me understand *why* I'm here—and find a meaningful way to use whatever time I have left."

Pets Point the Way in Our Search For Meaning

LaVonne's story touched my heart, because I know what it feels like to long for more meaning. I loved my job at Intuit, and I am incredibly grateful for the decade I spent there—but when I took the helm at Humane Society Silicon Valley, I felt like I had found a deeper purpose. The job wasn't easy at first. I faced hurdles and hit stumbling blocks when I tried to overhaul some aspects of the shelter. Meaningful work isn't stress-free, nor is it a path to perpetual bliss. But it leads to something better: It makes you feel like your life matters, and that confers a nourishing sense of well-being. In some small way, you're making a difference.

When it comes down to it, meaning is what nearly all of us crave. When American Express conducted a study looking at Americans' views of what makes a successful life, being healthy ranked first, but right behind that were a whole slew of concepts that correlate with meaning; finding time for the important things in life, having a good relationship or marriage, having a job you love, and making time to pursue passions and interests all ranked in the top seven most important aspects of success. Of the twenty-two items listed, having a lot of money ranked twentieth. After years of placing a high priority on wealth, many of us seem to have come to the same conclusion as Viktor Frankl, psychiatrist, Holocaust survivor, and author of *Man's Search for Meaning*: "Life is never made unbearable by circumstances but only by lack of meaning and purpose."

In our Mutual Rescue stories, varied as people's individual experiences are, a common thread emerged that I find truly extraordinary: In case after case, people who became more stable or happier or healthier after rescuing an animal went on to do something good in the world. It's the kind of outcome I wouldn't have noticed without soliciting hundreds of stories all at once. But hearing the various iterations of the same theme convinced me that the "rescue effect" is real. Adopting a shelter animal often opens humans' hearts and minds and brings their highest nature to the fore; they become more generous, kinder, and more giving. Many grow into people who care deeply about the state of the world and their fellow inhabitants on planet Earth.

Sixteen-year-old Grace Briden, who endured hours of fear and uncertainty in a classroom during the Marjory Stoneman Douglas shooting, ended up getting her family dog, Duncan, certified as a therapy animal, so she could help others the way the comfort dogs at school helped her in the weeks and months after the tragedy. "After I had him certified, I brought him to school with me and watched him comfort other students the way Karma comforted me," says Grace. "After the shooting it became important to me to do something good in the world."

Several years after the tiny kitten he named Scout crawled out from under a bush and saved his life, army veteran and PTSD sufferer Josh Marino returned to grad school, where he earned a master's degree in clinical rehab and mental health counseling so he could work with other veterans. "It was an extreme honor to wear the uniform of the U.S. military," he says. "By working with veterans who need the kind of help I did, I feel like I'm still serving and doing my part."

Motivated by his own weight loss after adopting Peety, Eric O'Grey left his job selling appliances and became director of philanthropy for the Physicians Committee for Responsible Medicine, an organization focused on preventing disease through plant-based diets and ending the cruel use of animals in medical studies. "Animal welfare is important to me, and I want people to know it's never too late to turn their health around," he says.

Many people who feel better after adopting a pet decide to put their efforts toward animal welfare, with the explicit hope that by helping animals, they'll also help people.

Nora Delaney was so inspired by the ability of her rescue dog, Max, to understand what she needed during her recovery from her umpteenth surgery, that she started a nonprofit fund-raiser, called Dining 4 Animals; friends attend a potluck dinner and donate the money they would have spent at a restaurant to local animal shelters. In eighteen months, she raised nearly $40,000.

Lis Phelps, whose cat, Ishtar, was her best friend and emotional support when she was broke, lonely, and unsure of what to do with her life, began fostering kittens for Kansas City Pet Project once her life became more stable. "I've helped a number of scrawny kittens go to their forever home," she says. "It's my way of passing along the love I got from Ishtar."

And after her dog, Prince, passed, Gemma Hunt knew she had to do something to help his legacy live on. So she began helping people train difficult dogs, and she and her husband, Darren, adopted two "unadoptable" dogs of their own. "I know how much difference a difficult dog can make in your life," she says. "To honor Prince, I've devoted my life to the animals that everyone else has given up on."

Philanthropic work is the ultimate act of faith—faith that what we do matters, that our actions can be used for good, that one individual can make a difference in the world. When people are moved to take that leap, the underlying force that propels their ability to act altruistically feels like something holy. And regardless of whether you believe in God or not, doing good in the world requires faith in the eternal existence and power of love.

As the Dalai Lama pointed out in an op-ed in the *New York Times*, "Selflessness and joy are intertwined. The more we are one with the rest of humanity, the better we feel."

Unfortunately, we live in era in which that feeling of "oneness" is becoming more elusive. As technology has transformed our lives—eliminating careers, eroding our ability to truly talk to one another and share deeply of ourselves, and dividing us into ideological bubbles that can drive a wedge between friends, neighbors, and family—it has diminished our sense of community, an important facet of meaning. But animals, as we've revealed throughout the book, can bridge the gap and unite even total strangers. And they can play an important role in other aspects of meaning as well.

In her book *The Power of Meaning*, positive psychology expert Emily Esfahani Smith identifies four pillars of meaning: a feeling of belonging, bonding, and love; having a sense of purpose by committing your time to something worthwhile; developing a life story, or narrative, that helps you understand yourself and the world; and experiencing moments of transcendence that make you feel connected to something larger than yourself. "These four qualities are part of the definitions of meaning that began with Aristotle and have been echoed by philosophers, psychologists, Buddhists, and filmmakers ever since," she told us. "Pets can potentially play a role in each of the four pillars. Their companionship and love provides a sense of belonging. The caretaking they require can be a source of purpose. They help you build a life narrative—as a 'dog person' or a 'cat person' or someone who cares about animal welfare. And bonding with another species can offer moments of transcendence."

Without at least one of those pillars, we're more likely to feel alienated, alone, and unfulfilled. With them, we can begin to find an answer to the ineffable question, "Why am I here?" And developing a close relationship with an animal, or in some cases, *many* animals, can be the experience that points us in the right direction.

How Fifty-Five Feral Cats Helped One Man Discover His Purpose

In 1995, Andrew Bloomfield was in his early thirties and had been a struggling screenwriter in Hollywood for several years when, after a period of homelessness, he moved into a bungalow with two friends. The bungalow's backyard was so overgrown with palm fronds, ivy, and old trees it looked like an Amazonian rainforest, and it was home to a large colony of feral cats and vulnerable kittens. At night, the coyotes and raccoons inevitably converged on the yard to prey on the tiny newborns. "At first I figured this was nature at work and none of my business," he says.

Then one day he walked out back and saw eight members of the colony sitting in a perfect semicircle around a dead kitten. "These weren't stray housecats. They were born in the wild, so they usually bolted when a human was around, and they never made eye contact. But this day, they just sat there calmly and looked back and forth between the kitten and me. They held my gaze. I don't know how to describe it except to say that I felt like I was being called to help," he says. "So I did."

Andrew began feeding the cats, and every night, he would sit in a chair in the backyard to keep predators away. "At first, none of the cats came near me, but as weeks turned to months they began to emerge from the shadows and sit with me," he says. "I started recognizing individual cats, naming each in order to keep track of them, and coming to appreciate their personalities and idiosyncrasies. In time, more than fifty cats emerged," he says. "For a while, I resisted neutering the cats because I thought I'd be interfering with the natural cycle of life, but the more I bonded with them, the more devastated I felt about not being able to protect all the newborns, despite my efforts. I finally reached a point where I couldn't stand one more puffball being carried away, so I started catching the colony members a few at a time and having them spayed and neutered."

What began as a project to fill his time became a passion. Andrew cared for the cats for more than twenty years—taking them to the vet to treat viruses, wounds, and abscesses, bringing orphaned littermates inside, giving them all the shelter of his love. He wrote a 2016 book about the experience, *Call of the Cats: What I Learned about Life and Love from a Feral Colony*. "In our culture, we're losing the ability to love and care for one another—and I probably would have been that way, too, if my career had been successful," he told us. "But the cats broke open my heart. My love affair with the colony challenged my ideas of love and family. They awoke in me the impulse to love and protect, and gave me a sense of worthiness. They made me more sensitive to the beauty and ingeniousness of nature, more able to find magic in small moments."

Most in the colony lived well beyond the expected life span of feral cats and died natural deaths from old age, rather than being victims of predators. But by now there are just a handful left. The passing of each and every cat was bittersweet, and some felines' deaths left a void in Andrew's heart that brings him pain to this day. But the experience was also the most profound of his life. "I thought I was destined for screenwriting greatness. Instead, a colony of feral cats adopted me and offered me a life filled with meaning and purpose beyond my unrealized Hollywood dreams."

Animals Present an Opportunity to Connect With the Ephemeral

I believe that companion animals were put on this earth for a reason: to help humans open their minds and hearts, as the feral colony did Andrew's. Nearly all of our Mutual Rescue participants talked about the way their animals had, as Andrew says, "cracked open" their hearts—and not long ago, I received a note from Susannah Greenwood, a frequent participant in our Doggy Day Out program (in which people come to the shelter and take a rescue dog on an outing for a few hours or a whole day) that revealed that even fleeting relationships with rescue animals can do the same. She wrote, "I love my three-legged rescue cats with all my heart, but these dogs and this program really are able to somehow fulfill a totally undiscovered part of my heart. Perhaps they are even an extension of it, allowing my heart to grow bigger with each outing."

Rescue animals can also, if we're open to it, reacquaint us with a spiritual world that we *Homo sapiens*, with our big, rational prefrontal cortexes, increasingly overlook, dismiss, or disregard. Faith can be a loaded word, but I think of it in the simplest form: belief that love is an entity that exists in and around us. I'm convinced that love is always waiting to flow through us, but we have to be receptive to it and attuned to its frequency; heartache, grief, addiction, and pain create static in that frequency, making it difficult to access—but rescuing an animal is one way to reset the dials, unclog the channel, and restore love's curative flow. John Ortberg, senior pastor at Menlo Church in Menlo Park, California, puts it this way: "We seem to be wired for connecting with animals. Having a creature to hold and love can make the peace of God real to us."

Our connection with our pets can be both concrete and mystical, though most of us pay attention only to the former. Those relationships are meaningful even if you don't believe there's anything more to it than petting, feeding, loving, and snuggling. But the creatures that drink from the toilet bowl and cough up blobs of fur at two a.m. also offer us a chance to glimpse life's mystery. After living alongside us for thousands of years, our companion animals have developed not only an affinity for mankind but also a sensitivity to what we're thinking and feeling that allows them, in many cases, to feel less like pets and more like fellow travelers on a shared journey.

The idea of an indefinable link between humans and animals shows up in serendipitous experiences like Bridget Keenan's, who was wooed by a rescue cat named Keenan just days after her beloved older sister, Mary, died. Even now, she shakes her head in wonder when she thinks about. "I mean, how did that happen?" she asks. "What are the chances?"

Mindy Beeler, whose one-eyed cat, Dorian, helped her cope with her grief after her mother took her own life, talks about her intense connection with Dorian in even more explicit terms. "I've had two different psychics tell me that Dorian and I knew each other in a previous life," she says. "I've never been one to believe those things, but it gives me chills sometimes when I look in his eye. It's like we know what the other one is thinking. It sounds crazy, but it happens all the time, and there's really no rational way to explain it."

Likewise, Brian and Kim Rose perceive a link between their dog, Lana, and their lost daughter, Aria. "Lana is 2.5 years old—about the same age Aria would be if she had lived," says Kim. "When you say 'Aria,' her ears perk up. One day, I said, 'Where's Aria?' and Lana ran over to the counter where Aria's picture was sitting. We do genuinely think that somehow, some way, Lana knows who Aria is. Maybe they even crossed paths somehow, in a way we don't understand. Last year for Father's Day I commissioned an artist to draw a picture of Aria sleeping, with Lana cuddled around her. It brings us great comfort. That's how Brian and I envision the two of them. Two parts of one whole."

Love is powerful—and, for me, it's not a stretch to believe that those deep, wordless relationships can transcend time and space, keeping us securely bound together, even if the precise explanation for how it happens is beyond our comprehension. It brings to mind a story I read about Bobby, a collie mix who became an international sensation in the 1920s. His owners, a couple who lived in Silverton, Oregon, were vacationing in Indiana when Bobby was lost. They looked for him everywhere. Finally, admitting he was gone for good, they headed home. Six months later, they woke up one morning, and there was Bobby, wagging his tail happily. Because the story was so improbable, Oregon Humane Society fact-checked the couple's story. They interviewed dozens of people from Indiana to Oregon, eventually reconstructing a reasonable approximation of Bobby's 2,800-mile odyssey.

In his book *One Mind*, Larry Dossey, MD, hypothesizes that Bobby was able to "home," pigeonlike, because he and his owners, and all of us who share this planet, are also part of a larger single mind; through that universal mind, Dr. Dossey says, the couple and Bobby were able to communicate, even though neither was consciously aware of it.

I've heard way too many stories from people who believe their animals know what they're thinking to dismiss this out of hand. And a second part of Dossey's premise I find even more credible. He says the distant sharing of knowledge is nearly always associated with love, caring, and compassion. I've seen the power of mutual love and fidelity between pets and people. I know it can be a source of strength for both species, giving each what they need to survive. And I know that the bond we create contains the power of infinite possibility.

A Pet's Affection Sets Love Free and Sends It Rippling Ever Outward

Pets are more than companions. They're characters in our life stories, adding color and texture to the narrative of our days. Large or small, short-haired or long, outgoing or reserved, rescue animals add richness and depth by filling our lives with laughter, frustration, delight, surprise, silliness, and heartache.

Once we've loved a pet, and absorbed their love for us, we're never the same. By winning us over, these endearing, willful creatures unleash our ability to feel compassion—the life-giving pulse at the center of meaning. Love, like other positive emotions, literally changes your mind, says Barbara Fredrickson, PhD, director of the University of North Carolina's Positive Emotions and Psychophysiology Lab. In her book *Love 2.0: Creating Happiness and Health in Moments of Connection,* she writes, "While infused with love you see fewer distinctions between you and others. Indeed, your ability to see others—really *see* them, wholeheartedly—springs open. Love can even give you a palpable sense of oneness and connection, a transcendence that makes you feel part of something far larger than yourself."

Animal-inspired compassion can take astonishing forms. Think of Andrew Bloomfield and his colony of feral cats. Then there's Carol Guzy, a four-time Pulitzer Prize–winning photojournalist, who has traveled from Haiti to Sierra Leone to Kosovo capturing gripping images of human suffering, heartbreak, and redemption. While she was in New Orleans covering Hurricane Katrina, she was so distraught by all the homeless animals left behind that she took a twelve-month leave of absence from the *Washington Post* to document their plight. Near the end of her time in New Orleans, she met the last orphan puppy at the Best Friends Animal Society's temporary shelter. The puppy's pregnant mother had consumed water contaminated with the storm's toxic runoff, affecting her offspring's development. "She was tiny and had tremors and couldn't walk because her back legs were weak and her front paws were deformed and turned inward," recalls Carol. "But it was obvious the instant I met her that inside her twisted body was a truly radiant spirit."

Carol adopted the little dog and named her Trixie. She did hours of hydrotherapy with her new dog to strengthen her muscles. "Trixie walked like Charlie Chaplin, but she was unstoppable. She was just bubbling over with unbridled joy. Everyone who met her fell in love with her. My mother was in a nursing home, and I'd take Trixie to visit all the residents. There's not a single person who didn't walk away changed by her huge heart and presence. She was the only source of joy for some of those older people."

Heartbreakingly, Trixie's neurological issues caught up with her, and she passed away less than six years after Carol brought her home. Carol had a memorial for Trixie at Best Friends' cemetery in Utah's Red Rock Canyon. It was a sunny, still day as they began the solemn Native American ceremony. Then the wind started to blow, and the hundreds of wind chimes hanging in the cemetery nearly drowned out the performers' chants. "My friend who works at the cemetery looked at me with her eyes wide and said, 'I've never seen that happen before. It's Trixie. She's here.' The moment the ceremony was over, the wind stopped," recalls Carol. "Losing Trixie was extremely difficult, but I share her story as much as I can because she was such a beacon of hope. She was broken. But we're all broken in some way—and she demonstrated every day how you don't need to let your brokenness define you. I still can't talk about her without crying. She was like a little angel walking on earth."

Our love for our pets can transform who we are and reveal who we are. In 2014, singer-songwriter Fiona Apple captured this idea eloquently in a letter she wrote to her fans, explaining why she was canceling the South American leg of her world tour. She wrote, in part:

> I have a dog, Janet, and she's been ill for about 2 years now, as a tumor has been idling in her chest, growing ever so slowly. She's almost 14 years old now. I got her when she was 4 months old. I was 21 back then—an adult, officially—and she was my kid. She is a pit bull, and was found in Echo Park, with a rope around her neck, and bites all over her ears and face. She was the one the dogfighters use to puff up the confidence of the contenders. She's almost 14 and I've never seen her start a fight, or bite, or even growl, so I can understand why they chose her for that awful role. She's a pacifist...
>
> She is my best friend, and my mother, and my daughter, my benefactor, and she's the one who taught me what love is...I know she is coming close to the time where she will stop being a dog and start instead to be part of everything. She'll be in the wind, and in the soil, and the snow, and in me, wherever I go. I just can't leave her now, please understand. If I go away again, I'm afraid she'll die and I won't have the honor of singing her to sleep, of escorting her out.
>
> Sometimes it takes me 20 minutes just to decide what socks to wear to bed.
>
> But this decision was instant.
>
> These are the choices we make, which define us. I will not be the woman who puts her career ahead of love & friendship. I am the woman who stays home, baking tilapia for my dearest, oldest friend. And helps her be comfortable & comforted & safe & important...
>
> So I am staying home, and I am listening to her snore and wheeze, and I am reveling in the swampiest, most awful breath that ever emanated from an angel. And I'm asking for your blessing.

Fiona's love for Janet is so real and palpable that I can imagine it makes the millions of people who've read the letter feel it, too—and, as a result, elevate all of us. That's why it's a mistake to see compassion for animals and compassion for humans as opposing agendas. It's not an either/or scenario. Loving our pets and promoting animal welfare can nurture and heighten our ability to care for and love our own species. Empathy isn't a zero-sum game.

This quote from Confucius expresses why rescue pets can be vectors of love that can help change the world: "To put our world in order we must first put our nation in order; to put our nation in order we must first put our community in order; to put our community in order, we must first put our family in order; to put our family in order we must first cultivate our personal life; we must first open our hearts." And one way to open our hearts is by adopting a homeless animal. As they wriggle their way into our affections, they give us the opportunity to practice and perfect our ability to be more fully, openly, fearlessly, compassionately human. They give us the opportunity to grow and evolve, to hope and heal. And they give us the opportunity to be wellsprings of love for one another.

Which is why, if rescue animals could talk to us, I think they'd say two things: The first is "Thank you."

The second: "*You're welcome.*"

About Mutual Rescue

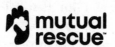

Follow us on Facebook, Twitter,
Instagram, and YouTube

VISIT MUTUALRESCUE.ORG TO:

Watch and Share Films—Several of the stories in this book are compelling short films. Grab a box of tissues and then share the films with friends on social media!

Watch and Share Tribute Montages—For anyone who has loved and lost a pet, the photography, poetry, and music of these films provide comfort by reaffirming the enduring bonds between animals and people.

Sign Up for Updates—Be the first to hear news about Mutual Rescue and receive alerts for new film releases.

Submit Your Story—Have your own story of mutual rescue? We'd love to hear about it for possible consideration in an upcoming film or book.

Find a Doggy Day Out Program—A shelter dog in your community wants to go on an outing with you. Enjoy a fun doggy date while helping an animal in need. Locate a program and get started!

Adopt an Animal—Inspired to add a pet to your family? There are millions of homeless animals waiting to find their forever families.

Find a Local Shelter or Rescue Organization—Want to get more involved? Find a local shelter or rescue organization and become a volunteer or donor.

Resources for Shelters and Rescue Organizations:

Host a Mutual Rescue Film Festival—Mutual Rescue films are available for free to shelters and rescue organizations to use offline for fund-raising and to drive community awareness and engagement.

Start a Doggy Day Out Program—If you're involved with a shelter or rescue organization that would love to start a program, download our free toolkit. Already have a program at your shelter? Let us know so we can list it in our directory.

For Corporations:

Discover the Benefits of Sponsorship—Interested in partnering with a brand that is exciting, engaging, and emotional? Let's talk!

Watch Our Story—Learn more about Mutual Rescue and the power of our brand to improve the lives of both humans and animals.

SHELTERS AND RESCUE ORGANIZATIONS
REFERENCED IN THE BOOK

100+ Abandoned Dogs of Everglades Florida Rescue — Wilton Manors, Florida

Angels Among Us — Alpharetta, Georgia

Animal Friends Rescue Project — Pacific Grove, California

Animal Rescue League of Berks County — Birdsboro, Pennsylvania

Animal Rescue League of El Paso — El Paso, Texas

ASPCA Adoption Center in NYC — New York, New York

Bath Dogs and Cats Home — Bath, England

Best Friends Animal Society — Kanab, Utah, and Mission Hills, California

Central Missouri Humane Society — Columbia, Missouri

Foothills Animal Shelter — Golden, Colorado

Fort Riley Stray Animal Shelter — Fort Riley, Kansas

Hog Haven Farm — Deer Trail, Colorado

Humane Society of Boulder Valley — Boulder, Colorado

Humane Society of Broward County — Fort Lauderdale, Florida

Humane Society of the Pikes Peak Region — Colorado Springs, Colorado

Humane Society Silicon Valley — Milpitas, California

Humane Society of Sonoma County — Santa Rosa, California

Joint Animal Services of Thurston County — Olympia, Washington

Kansas City Pet Project — Kansas City, Missouri

Kitty Bungalow-Charm School for Wayward Cats — Los Angeles, California

Nate's Honor Animal Rescue — Bradenton, Florida

Nevada Humane Society — Carson City, Nevada

New Beginnings for Cats	Bourbonnais, Illinois
Nine Lives Foundation	Redwood City, California
Oregon Humane Society	Portland, Oregon
Palm Beach County Animal Care and Control	West Palm Beach, Florida
Paws and Warriors	Bradenton, Florida
Paws in the City	Dallas, Texas
Puppy Rescue Mission	Celina, Texas
Seattle Humane Society	Bellevue, Washington
San Francisco Animal Care & Control	San Francisco, California
San Francisco SPCA	San Francisco, California
Throw Away Dogs Project	Huntingdon Valley, Pennsylvania

RESCUE THERAPY PROGRAMS REFERENCED IN THE BOOK

Animal Assisted Therapy Programs of Colorado	Lakewood, Colorado
Eponicity	La Fortuna, Costa Rica
Equine Healing Collaborative	Carmel, California
Inmates Nursing Kittens	Carson City, Nevada
Pet Partners	Bellevue, Washington
Prison Pet Partnership	Gig Harbor, Washington

Acknowledgments

Loving the animals that share our homes is easy. Understanding what that love does for us is more complex. We're grateful to every person who is mentioned in these pages for helping us peer deeply into this familiar human experience and reveal the hidden gems inside the marvelous, ordinary mystery of the human–animal bond. To those who shared their personal stories, thank you for opening your lives and hearts, for your patience with our probing questions, and for having the courage to reflect candidly on the meaningful ways your relationships with your animals have enriched your lives. To the researchers around the world whose superb work is providing a deeper understanding of why so many of us are besotted with (and often beholden to) our pets, your generosity with your time, insights, and scientific wisdom was deeply appreciated.

We're indebted to several people in particular: Bonnie Solow, Carol's literary agent and Ginny's dear friend, who had the brilliant insight to bring us together to collaborate on this project; Karen Murgolo at Grand Central Life & Style, who saw the potential in an animal book that contained stories and science and whose sharp edits and observant questions made this manuscript much better; the entire team at Grand Central Life & Style for their talents in ensuring the book's success; and Lorrie Sprain, whose organizational skills and attention to administrative details made delivering the final manuscript possible.

Acknowledgments from Carol:

I frequently say "it takes a village," and I have seen that notion powerfully enacted during the creation of Mutual Rescue. I am deeply grateful to the many contributors who have partnered with me to bring this book, the Mutual Rescue films, and the overall initiative to life: My extraordinarily talented writing collaborator, Ginny Graves, for your gift of creating compelling narratives and instinctively knowing the right amount of "heart" and "head" to blend together to engage readers. It's been a true delight and privilege to collaborate with you to create this manuscript. Marci Shimoff, for recognizing that Mutual Rescue had the potential to become a book and for graciously opening your Rolodex on my behalf to make it happen. Bonnie Solow for believing in me and Mutual Rescue and nurturing our professional relationship long before it was apparent I'd be brave enough to write a book. Emily Charnes, Ginny Neal, and Diann Lawson for cheering me on throughout the writing process and serving as reliable and thoughtful sounding boards.

This book began with the Mutual Rescue films, and those would never have happened without an enormous cast of characters, to each of whom I'm indebted.

David Whitman for breathing magic into the idea that "helping animals helps people," designing and orchestrating the call for stories, and serving as executive producer of the Mutual Rescue films—and Sally Hazard Bourgoin for having the foresight to introduce me to him. Doug Scott and the team at Advocate Creative for your brilliant cinematography and talent for authentic storytelling. Eric O'Grey for being the first to trust us with your story; without you and Peety, Mutual Rescue would not be where it is today. Joel and Heidi Roberts for helping me gracefully articulate the essence of Mutual Rescue. Timi and John M. Sobrato for being the first to believe and invest in this concept. Sue and John Diekman, Willow, N & P, the Nikki and Rich Beyer family, Dan and Kathy McCranie, Blythe Jack and Bob Rider, Derk Hunter, Kingsley Jack Dr. David Haworth and the team at PetSmart Charities, and Mary Ippoliti-Smith and the team at Maddie's Fund for your generous support that has allowed us to continue making films and building the brand. Steve Kirton and the team at Circa Healthcare for believing in this work so early on and providing not only your time and talent but also making connections on our behalf. Jeanni Stevens for making the introduction to Steve.

Stephanie Ladeira, Joanne Jacobs, Finn Dowling, Sandy Mallalieu, and Stephanie Warne for the talent, time, and heart you give to building this brand and taking on yet another project when your plates are already overfull. All of our Mutual Rescue film subjects, judges, and story evaluators, as well as the artists and contributors to our montage films, I am deeply humbled by your willingness to share your stories, time, and expertise with us. Michelle Tennant Nicholson and Wasabi Publicity, Tom Cohen and Animal Welfare Media, Chris Raniere and 46Mile, David Tenzer, Tracy Randall and Sally Abel and Fenwick & West, David Gilmour, Bouree Nordin, Jenifer Willig and Hive, Barbara Sauceda, Richard Eveleigh, and Caitlin Daly for deploying your talents into this initiative. And to all of the shelters with Doggy Day Out programs and whose animals are featured in Mutual Rescue films and stories, it's an honor and a privilege to be highlighting your work and impact.

In addition, Mutual Rescue exists because of the incredible support of so many people associated with Humane Society Silicon Valley, to which I am deeply grateful: Sue Diekman, board chair when Mutual Rescue launched, for your unbridled enthusiasm and all of your support over the years. Kurt Krukenberg, HSSV's current board chair, for continuing that same level of support and enthusiasm, along with our entire board of directors. Thank you for your unwavering belief in me and HSSV's mission. Mike for changing the course of my career and being my rock during the initial years at HSSV. I also want to thank: Dr. Cristie Kamiya, Candice Balmaceda, Yvonne Saucedo, and Jeanne Wu for being on this professional journey with me. Susanne Kogut and the Petco Foundation and Petco teams for their ongoing support. And to all of the employees, volunteers, and donors at HSSV, thank you for all you do day in and day out to support and care for homeless animals and find them loving forever families.

To my colleagues and mentors from Intuit, the lessons learned and insights gleaned from you over the years are woven throughout both Mutual Rescue and Humane Society Silicon Valley. Thank you for playing such a significant role in shaping me into the leader I am today.

And most important, I am grateful for all of the people who love and bless me by being "secure anchors" and "safe havens" in my life: the Norcal Gal Pals, the YML Miracle Sisters and my YML Heart Group, Bahar Zadeh, and my friends from Conestoga, Dickinson College, Harvard Business School, and Menlo Church. Jan Schroeder for over twenty years of thoughtful perspective, guidance, and love. And to my family: my sister and brother-in-law, Barb and Bob, and my nieces, Amelia and Julia, for always being there and providing me with a deep sense of family; my mother, Sally, and brother, Fred, for our shared love of felines, and my father, Fred, who will always be a part of me. And of course, my beloved four-legged furry family members, Tess, Bode, and Herbie, who light up my life with their companionship and silliness every single day.

Acknowledgments from Ginny:

I was on a local trail with my friend Bonnie Solow and our rowdy puppies, Daisy and Tullah, when she asked me if I'd be interested in working on a book about rescue animals. So launched an eighteen-month journey into the enthralling, uplifting, extraordinary universe of the human-animal bond—an experience that changed the way I look at both animals and people and the power those relationships have to shape and enrich our everyday lives. My heartfelt thanks to the brilliant Carol Novello, whose comprehensive philosophy about the power of the human-animal bond is both eye-opening and inspiring—and has the capacity to change the world. I'm grateful to you for bringing me along on this adventure and making this project a delight from start to finish.

I'm also indebted to the kindred spirits who, blessedly, always trudge along beside me: Susan Cronk, Diane Phillips, and Carol Lieske Williams; to my smart, funny, always-there writer's group—Laura Hilgers, Barbara Graham, Kathy Ellison and Ronnie Cohen; to my beloved Belvidere Park crew (you know who you are); and to my mom, Marlene Graves, whose voice on the other end of the phone is the thing I most look forward to every morning.

My infatuation with animals began when I was five and my parents gave me a book about dogs for Christmas—a love affair that has grown with every cat and dog whose fur has blanketed my sofa. I'm grateful to you, Mom and Dad, for kindling my passion for animals, and to my husband, Gordon, for abetting it—for being the guy who plays fetch on the street at dawn so I can start writing, always has poop bags on hand, and patiently agrees that, yes, we *should* adopt a puppy, even though we have two dogs already. Your steadfast support is the reason I'm able to do what I do. That sweet legacy lives in our sons, Will and Griffin, who learned early on how to love cats and dogs and have grown into kind and empathetic young men. May the word "family" always include a haphazard assortment of furry beasts.

Finally, to our three adoring canines, Kiki, Lola, and Daisy, who were rarely out of petting range for the duration of this project: Thank you for being so patient. Who wants to go for a hike?

Sources

Introduction

ASPCA, "Shelter Intake and Surrender" (https://www.aspca.org/animal-homeless ness/shelter-intake-and-surrender/pet-statistics).

National Philanthropic Trust, "Charitable Giving Statistics" (https://www.nptrust .org/philanthropic-resources/charitable-giving-statistics).

Charity Navigator, "Giving Statistics, Giving USA 2018, The Annual Report on Philan-thropy" (https://www.charitynavigator.org/index.cfm?bay=content.view&cpid=42).

National Institute of Mental Health, "Prevalence of Major Depressive Episode Among Adults," 2016 (https://www.nimh.nih.gov/health/statistics/major-dep ression.shtml).

U.S. Department of Veterans Affairs, *PTSD: National Center for PTSD,* "How Common Is PTSD" (https://www.ptsd.va.gov/public/ptsd-overview/basics/how -common-is-ptsd.asp).

Centers for Disease Control and Prevention, CDC Newsroom, "More than 29 mil-lion Americans have diabetes; 1 in 4 doesn't know it" (https://www.cdc.gov/ media/releases/2014/p0610-diabetes-report.html).

Centers for Disease Control and Prevention, *Overweight & Obesity,* "Adult Obesity Facts" (https://www.cdc.gov/obesity/data/adult.html).

HABRI Human Animal Bond Research Institute, *2014 Physician Survey,* "Pets and Health" (https://habri.org/2014-physician-survey).

Harvard Second Generation Study, *Study of Adult Development,* "History of the Study" (http://www.adultdevelopmentstudy.org/grantandglueckstudy).

"The Two Pillars of Happiness," *Medium,* October 25, 2015. (https://medium.com/ @OnFormForever/the-two-pillars-of-happiness-9dcb5a72e276).

SECTION I: HEART

Chapter 1: Finding Courage

Brené Brown, *I Thought It Was Just Me: Women Reclaiming Power and Courage in a Culture of Shame* (Gotham, 2007).

John Bowlby, *Attachment and Loss: Volume 1—Attachment* and *Volume 2—Separation* (Basic Books, 1969, 1982).

Lauren A. O'Connell, Hans A. Hofmann, "Evolution of a Vertebrate Social Decision-Making Network," *Science* 336, no. 6085 (June 1, 2012): 1154–1157.

Sigal Zilcha-Mano, Mario Mikulincer, Phillip R. Shaver, "An attachment perspective on human-pet relationships: Conceptualization and assessment of pet attachment orientations," *Journal of Research in Personality* 45, no. 4 (August 2011): 345–357.

Connect@BreneBrown email entitled "What's New on BreneBrown.com" dated November 9, 2017.

National Coalition Against Domestic Violence, "Statistics." (https://ncadv.org/statistics)

Mindy Mechanic, Terri Weaver, and Patricia Resick, "Mental Health Consequences of Intimate Partner Abuse: A Multidimensional Assessment of Four Different Forms of Abuse," *Violence Against Women* 14 no. 6 (June 2008): 634-654.

Amy Fitzgerald, "'They Gave Me a Reason to Live': The protective effects of companion animals on the suicidality of abused women," *Humanity & Society* 31 no. 4 (November 2007): 355-378.

For a searchable database of animal rescue facilities that offer shelter for the pets of victims of domestic violence, go to awionline.org/safehavens. Additional resources can also be found at safeplaceforpets.org and redrover.org.

Tori DeAngelis, "The Two Faces of Oxytocin," *American Psychological Association*, February 2008. (http://www.apa.org/monitor/feb08/oxytocin.aspx).

Humane Society of the United States, news release, "Clark, Ros-Lehtinen Bill Protects Domestic Violence Victims and Pets," March 5, 2015. (http://www.humanesociety.org/news/press_releases/2015/03/domestic-violence-and-pets-030515.html).

Chapter 2: Building Trust

"Pema Chodron and Jack Kornfield Talk 'The Wondrous Path of Difficulties,'" Lion's Roar, October 15, 2017. (https://www.lionsroar.com/the-wondrous-path-of-difficulties/).

Carlos A. Driscoll, Marilyn Menotti-Raymond, Alfred L. Roca, Karsten Hupe, Warren E. Johnson, Eli Geffen, Eric Harley, Miguel Delibes, Dominique Pontier, Andrew C. Kitchener, Nobuyuki Yamaguchi, Stephen J. O'Brien, and David Macdonald, "The Near Eastern Origin of Cat Domestication," *Science* 317 no. 5837 (July 27, 2007): 519-523.

Carlos A. Driscoll, Juliet Clutton-Brock, Andrew C. Kitchener, and Stephen J. O'Brien, "The Taming of the Cat," *Scientific American*, 300, no. 6 (June 2009): 68-75

Melanie L. Glocker, Daniel D. Langleben, Kosha Ruparel, James W. Loughead, Ruben C. Gur, and Norbert Sachser, "Baby Schema in Infant Faces Induces Cuteness Perception and Motivation for Caretaking in Adults," *Ethology* 115, no. 3 (March 2009): 257–263.

Statista, The Statistics Portal, "Number of Cats in the United States from 2000 to 2017/2018" (https://www.statista.com/statistics/198102/cats-in-the-united-states-since-2000/).

Debi Grebenik and Focus on the Family, *Hope & Healing Through Animal-Assisted Therapy* (2015). (Booklet available at http://shop.focusonthefamily.ca/Parenting/Adoption/Hope-Healing-Through-Animal-Assisted-Therapy-Booklet.html.)

Sam Carr and Ben Rockett, "Fostering Secure Attachment: Experiences of Animal Companions in the Foster Home," *Attachment and Human Development* 19, no. 3 (June 2017): 259-277.

Stephanie Pappas, "Oxytocin: Facts About the 'Cuddle Hormone,'" *LiveScience*, June 4, 2015 (https://www.livescience.com/42198-what-is-oxytocin.html).

Paul Zak, et al., "Oxytocin Is Associated with Human Trustworthiness," *Hormones and Behavior* 48, no. 5 (December 2005): 522-527.

Chapter 3: Coping with Grief

C. S. Lewis, *A Grief Observed* (Faber and Faber, 1961).

Andrea Volpe, "Is Grief a Disease?" *The Atlantic*, November 16, 2016 (https://www.theatlantic.com/health/archive/2016/11/when-grief-never-ends/507752/).

Fran Schumer, "After a Death, the Pain That Doesn't Go Away," *New York Times*, September 28, 2009 (https://www.nytimes.com/2009/09/29/health/29grief.html).

Michael Shermer, "Five Fallacies of Grief: Debunking Psychological Stages," *Scientific American*, November 1, 2008 (https://www.scientificamerican.com/article/five-fallacies-of-grief/).

Anna Milberg and Maria Friedrichsen, "Attachment Figures When Death Is Approaching: A Study Applying Attachment Theory to Adult Patients' and Family Members' Experiences during Palliative Care at Home," *Supportive Cancer Care* 25, no. 7 (February 2017): 2267–2274.

Deborah Custance and Jennifer Mayer, "Empathic-like Responding by Domestic Dogs (*Canis familiaris*) to Distress in Humans: An Exploratory Study," *Animal Cognition* 15, no. 5 (September 2012): 851–859.

Thomas Attig, *The Heart of Grief: Death and the Search for Lasting Love* (Oxford University Press, 2000).

Anne Lamott (https://www.goodreads.com/quotes/70759-you-will-lose-someone-you-can-t-live-without-and-your-heart). Used with email permission dated September 25, 2018, from Anne Lamott.

Chapter 4: Flourishing after Sorrow

Bill Moyers on Faith and Reason, "Bill Moyers and Pema Chödrön," August 4, 2006 (http://www.pbs.org/moyers/faithandreason/print/faithandreason107_print.html).

Michael Meehan, Bronwyn Massavelli, and Nancy Pachana, "Using Attachment Theory and Social Support Theory to Examine and Measure Pets as Sources of Social Support and Attachment Figures," *Anthrozoos*, 30, no. 2 (2017): 273–289.

Andrea Haffly, "Prison Pet Partnership Expands Its Reach," *The News Tribune*, April 20, 2016. (https://www.thenewstribune.com/news/local/community/gateway/g-news/article72888682.html).

Olivia DeGennaro, "Inmates Nursing Kittens Program Gives Both Felons and Felines New Lease on Life," News 4, May 12, 2016 (https://mynews4.com/news/local/inmates-nursing-kittens-program-gives-both-felons-and-felines-new-lease-on-life).

SECTION II: BODY

Chapter 5: Vitalizing Physical Health

Glenn N. Levine, Karen Allen, Lynne T. Braun, Hayley E. Christian, Erika Friedmann, Kathryn A. Taubert, Sue Ann Thomas, Deborah L. Wells, and Richard A. Lange, "Pet Ownership and Cardiovascular Risk: A Scientific Statement from the American Heart Association," *Circulation* 127, no. 23 (June11, 2013): 2353–2363.

HABRI (Human Animal Bond Research Institute), *2014 Physician Survey,* "Pets and Health" (https://habri.org/2014-physician-survey).

Centers for Disease Control and Prevention, National Center for Health Statistics, "Overweight and Obesity" (https://www.cdc.gov/nchs/fastats/obesity-overweight.htm).

Centers for Disease Control and Prevention, National Center for Health Statistics, "Exercise or Physical Activity" (https://www.cdc.gov/nchs/fastats/exercise.htm).

Centers for Disease Control and Prevention, "At a Glance 2016 Heart Disease and Stroke" (https://www.cdc.gov/chronicdisease/resources/publications/aag/pdf/2016/aag-heart-disease.pdf).

American Heart Association, "Heart Disease and Stroke Statistics 2017 At-a-Glance" (https://healthmetrics.heart.org/wp-content/uploads/2017/06/Heart-Disease-and-Stroke-Statistics-2017-ucm_491265.pdf).

E. Friedman, A. H. Katcher, J. J. Lynch, and S. A. Thomas, "Animal Companions and One-year Survival of Patients after Discharge from a Coronary Care Unit," *Public Health Reports*, 95, no. 4 (July–August 1980): 307–312.

Adnan I. Qureshi, Muhammad Zeeshan Memon, Gabriela Vazquez, M. Fareed, and K. Suri, "Cat Ownership and the Risk of Fatal Cardiovascular Diseases. Results from the second National Health and Nutrition Examination Study Mortality Follow-up Study," *Journal of Vascular and Interventional Neurology* 2, no. 1 (January 2009): 132–135.

Imala Ogechi, Kassandra Snook, Bionca M. Davis, Andrew R. Hansen, Fengqi Liu, and Jian Zhang, "Pet Ownership and the Risk of Dying from Cardiovascular

Disease among Adults without Major Chronic Medical Conditions," *High Blood Pressure & Cardiovascular Prevention*, 23, no. 3 (September 2016): 245–253.

Mwenya Mubanga, Liisa Byberg, Christoph Nowak, Agneta Egenvall, Patrik K. Magnusson, Erik Ingelsson, and Tove Fall, "Dog Ownership and the Risk of Cardiovascular Disease and Death—A Nationwide Cohort Study," *Scientific Reports* (https://www.nature.com/articles/s41598-017-16118-6).

HeartMath Institute, "A Boy and His Dog—Heart Rhythm Entrainment" (https://www.heartmath.com/inspire-a-change-of-heart/).

Fiona Macrae, "Dogs' Hearts Beat in Sync with their Owners Says Latest Study to Show Having a Pet Is Good for Keeping Healthy," DailyMail.com (http://www.dailymail.co.uk/sciencetech/article-3568690/Dogs-hearts-beat-sync-owners-says-latest-study-having-pet-good-keeping-healthy.html).

Rebecca A. Johnson and Richard L. Meadows, "Dog-walking: Motivation for Adherence to a Walking Program," *Clinical Nursing Research* 19, no. 4 (November 2010): 387–402.

Gukowska, M. Jankowski, S. Mukaddam-Daher, and S. M. McCann, "Oxytocin Is a Cardiovascular Hormone," *Brazilian Journal of Medical and Biological Research*, 33, no. 6 (June 2000): 625–633.

Chapter 6: Embracing Joy

Nicole K. Valtora, Mona Kanaan, Simon Gilbody, Sara Ronzi, and Barbara Hanratty, "Loneliness and Social Isolation as Risk Factors for Coronary Heart Disease and Stroke: Systematic Review and Meta-analysis of Longitudinal Observational Studies," *British Medical Journal*, 2016.

Julianne Holt-Lunstad, Timothy B. Smith, Mark Baker, Tyler Harris, and David Stephenson, "Loneliness and Social Isolation as Risk Factors for Mortality," *Perspectives on Psychological Science*, 102, no. 13 (March 2015): 227–237.

"U.K. Appoints a Minister for Loneliness," *New York Times*, January 17, 2018 (https://www.nytimes.com/2018/01/17/world/europe/uk-britain-loneliness.html).

Louise C. Hawkley and John T. Cacioppo, "Loneliness Matters: A Theoretical and Empirical Review of Consequences and Mechanisms," *Annals of Behavioral Medicine*, 40, No. 2 (October 2010) 218–227 (https://www.ncbi.nlm.nih.gov/pmc/articles/PMC3874845/).

Raheel Mushtaq, Sheik Shoib, Tabindah Shah, and Sahil Mushtaq, "Relationship between Loneliness, Psychiatric Disorders and Physical Health," *Journal of Clinical Diagnostic Research*, 8, no. 9 (September 2014) WE01-WE-04 (https://www.ncbi.nlm.nih.gov/pmc/articles/PMC4225959/).

G. Oscar Anderson, "Loneliness among Older Adults: A National Survey of Adults 45+," AARP Research, September 2010 (https://www.aarp.org/content/dam/aarp/research/surveys_statistics/general/2012/loneliness-2010.doi.10.26419%252Fres.00064.001.pdf).

Sean Coughlan, "Loneliness More Likely to Affect Young People," BBC News, April 10, 2018 (https://www.bbc.com/news/education-43711606).

Laignee Barron, "British People Are So Lonely That They Now Have a Minister for Loneliness," *TIME* magazine, January 18, 2018 (http://time.com/5107252/minister-for-loneliness-uk/).

Parya Saberi, et al., "Association between Dog Guardianship and HIV Clinical Outcomes," *Journal of the International Association of Providers of AIDS Care*, 13, no. 4 (July–August 2014): 300–304 (https://www.ncbi.nlm.nih.gov/pmc/articles/PMC3995900/).

Jitka Pikhartova, et al., "Does Owning a Pet Protect Older People against Loneliness?" *BMC Geriatrics*, 14, no. 106 (September 2014) (https://www.ncbi.nlm.nih.gov/pmc/articles/PMC4182770/).

Keri Black, "The Relationship between Companion Animals and Loneliness among Rural Adolescents," *Journal of Pediatric Nursing*, 27, no. 2 (April 2012): 103–112.

Marian R. Banks and William Banks, "The Effects of Animal-Assisted Therapy on Loneliness in an Elderly Population in Long-Term Care Facilities," *The Journals of Gerontology*, 57, no. 7 (July 2002): M428–M432.

Lisa Wood, Karen Martin, Hayley Christian, Andrea Nathan, Claire Lauritsen, Steve Houghton, Ichiro Kawachi, and Sandra McCune, "The Pet Factor—Companion Animals as a Conduit for Getting to Know People, Friendship Formation and Social Support," *PLOS One*, 10, no. 4 (April 2015) (http://journals.plos.org/plosone/article/file?id=10.1371/journal.pone.0122085&type=printable).

Chapter 7: Overcoming Illness and Injury

Michele L. Morrison, "Health Benefits of Animal-Assisted Interventions," *Complementary Health Practices Review*, 12, no. 1 (January 2007): 51–62 (http://journals.sagepub.com/doi/pdf/10.1177/1533210107302397).

Peggy Nepps, Charles Stewart, and Stephen Bruckno, "Animal Assisted Therapy: Effects on Stress, Mood and Pain," *The Journal of Lancaster General Hospital*, Summer 2011 (http://www.jlgh.org/Past-Issues/Volume-6—Issue-2/Animal-Assisted-Therapy.aspx).

Centers for Disease Control and Prevention, Chronic Disease Prevention and Health Promotion, "Chronic Disease Overview" (https://www.cdc.gov/chronicdisease/overview/index.htm).

National Health Council, "About Chronic Conditions" (http://www.nationalhealthcouncil.org/newsroom/about-chronic-conditions#1).

Amy McCullough, Ashleigh Ruehrdanz, and Molly Jenkins, "The Use of Dogs in Hospital Settings," HABRI Central, January 2016. (https://habricentral.org/resources/54871/download/hc_brief_dogsinhospitals20160115Access.pdf).

Hiroharu Kamioka, Shinpei Okada, Kiichiro Tsutani, et al., "Effectiveness of Animal-Assisted Therapy: A Systematic Review of Randomized Controlled Trials," *Complementary Therapies in Medicine*, 22, no. 2 (April 2014) 371-390 (http://

www.f.u-tokyo.ac.jp/~utdpm/2014%20Kamioka%20animal-assisted%20therapy %20CTM.pdf).

Michele L. Morrison, "Health Benefits of Animal-Assisted Interventions," *Journal of Evidence-Based Integrative Medicine* 12, no. 1 (January 1, 2007): 51–62

Centers for Disease Control and Prevention, Injury Prevention & Control, "Key Injury and Violence Data" (https://www.cdc.gov/injury/wisqars/overview/ key_data.html).

Taneal A. Wiseman, Kate Curtis, Mary Lam, and Kim Foster, "Incidence of Depression, Anxiety and Stress Following Traumatic Injury: A Longitudinal Study," *Scandinavian Journal of Trauma, Resuscitation and Emergency Medicine*, 23 (March 28, 2015) (https://www.ncbi.nlm.nih.gov/pmc/articles/PMC4389309/).

Hilde Myhren, Oivind Ekegerg, Kirsti Toien, Susanne Karlsson, and Olav Stokland, "Post-traumatic Stress, Anxiety and Depression Symptoms in Patients during the First Year Post Intensive Care Unit Discharge," *Critical Care*, 14, no. 1 (2010) R14 (https://www.ncbi.nlm.nih.gov/pmc/articles/PMC2875529/).

Friederike Range and Zsofia Viranyi, "Tracking the Evolutionary Origins of Dog-Human Cooperation: The 'Canine Cooperation Hypothesis,'" *Frontiers in Psychology,* 5 (January 2015) (https://www.frontiersin.org/articles/10.3389/ fpsyg.2014.01582/full).

Gregory S. Berns, Andrew M. Brooks, Mark Spivak, and Kerinne Levy, "Functional MRI in Awake Dogs Predicts Suitability for Assistance Work," *Scientific Reports*, 7 (March 2017).

John W. Pilley and Alliston K. Reid, "Border Collie Comprehends Object Names as Verbal Referents," *Behavioural Processes*, Febuary 2011: 184–195.

Pet Partners, email communication. March 7, 2018.

Megan M. Hosey, Janice Jaskulski, Stephen T. Wegener, Linda L. Chlan, and Dale M. Needham, "Animal-Assisted Intervention in the ICU: A Tool for Humanization," *Critical Care*, 22, no. 22 (February 2018) 1946–1948 (https://ccforum .biomedcentral.com/articles/10.1186/s13054-018-1946-8).

Rodrigo Cavallazzi, Mohamed Saad, and Paul E. Marik, "Delirium in the ICU: An Overview," *Annals of Intensive Care*, 2 (December 2012) (https://www.ncbi.nlm .nih.gov/pmc/articles/PMC3539890/).

Chapter 8: Recovering from Addiction

Anne Case and Angus Deaton, "Mortality and Morbidity in the 21st Century," *Brookings Papers on Economic Activity*, Spring 2017 (https://www.brookings.edu/ wp-content/uploads/2017/08/casetextsp17bpea.pdf).

Substance Abuse and Mental Health Services Administration, *Behavioral Health Trends in the United States: Results from the 2014 National Survey on Drug Use and Health.* (https://www.samhsa.gov/data/sites/default/files/NSDUH-FRR1-2014/ NSDUH-FRR1-2014.pdf).

Josh Katz, "The First Count of Fentanyl Deaths in 2016 Up 540% in Three Years," *New York Times*, September 2, 2017 (https://www.nytimes.com/interactive/2017/09/02/upshot/fentanyl-drug-overdose-deaths.html).

Centers for Disease Control, NCHS Data Brief No. 294, December 2017, "Drug Overdose Deaths in the United States, 1999–2016" (https://www.cdc.gov/nchs/data/databriefs/db294.pdf).

National Archives, Military Records, *Vietnam War U.S. Military Fatal Casualty Statistics* (https://www.archives.gov/research/military/vietnam-war/casualty-statistics).

Iraq Coalition Casualty Count, icasualties.org (http://icasualties.org/).

Center on Addiction, "Addiction by the Numbers" (https://www.centeronaddiction.org/).

National Institute of Drug Abuse, "Nationwide Trends" (https://www.drugabuse.gov/publications/drugfacts/nationwide-trends).

Partnership for Drug-Free Kids, "Survey: Ten Percent of American Adults Report Being in Recovery from Substance Abuse or Addiction" (https://drugfree.org/newsroom/news-item/survey-ten-percent-of-american-adults-report-being-in-recovery-from-substance-abuse-or-addiction/).

Hazelden Betty Ford Foundation, Research Update Butler Center for Research, "Animal-Assisted Therapy for Substance Use Disorders," July 2016 (https://www.hazeldenbettyford.org/articles/together/animal-assisted-healing-hope).

Dawn A. Marcus, Cheryl D. Bernstein, Janet M. Constantin, Frank A. Kunkel, Paula Breuer, and Raymond B. Hanlon, "Impact of Animal-Assisted Therapy for Outpatients with Fibromyalgia," *Pain Medicine*, 14, no. 1 (January 2013): 43–51 (https://www.ncbi.nlm.nih.gov/pmc/articles/PMC3666031/).

Canadian Centre on Substance Use and Addiction, *Life in Recovery from Addiction in Canada, Technical Report,* May 2017 (http://www.ccdus.ca/Resource%20Library/CCSA-Life-in-Recovery-from-Addiction-Report-2017-en.pdf).

Martin C. Wesley, Neresa B. Minatrea, and Joshua C. Watson, "Animal-Assisted Therapy in Treatment of Substance Dependence," *Anthrozoos*, 22, no. 2 (2009): 137–148 (https://www.tandfonline.com/doi/abs/10.2752/175303709X434167).

Lindsay Madden Ellsworth, Sarah Tragesser, and Ruth C. Newberry, "Interaction with Shelter Dogs Reduces Negative Affect of Adolescents in Substance Use Disorder Treatment," *Anthrozoos*, 29, no. 2 (May 2016): 247–262 (https://www.tandfonline.com/doi/abs/10.1080/08927936.2016.1152719).

SECTION III: MIND

Chapter 9: Cultivating Grit

Angela Duckworth, *Grit: The Power of Passion and Perseverance* (Scribner, 2016), 275.

Angela Duckworth, Christopher Peterson, Michael D. Matthews, and Dennis R. Kelly, "Grit: Perseverance and Passion for Long-Term Goals," *Journal of Personality and Social Psychology*, 92, no. 6 (July 2007): 1087–1101.

Angela L. Duckworth and Martin E. P. Seligman, "Self-Discipline Outdoes IQ in Predicting Academic Performance of Adolescents," *Psychological Science*, 16, no. 12 (December 2005): 939–944.

Angela L. Duckworth, Teri A. Kirby, Eli Tsukayama, et al., "Deliberate Practice Spells Success: Why Grittier Competitors Triumph at the National Spelling Bee," *Social Psychological and Personality Science*, 2, no. 2 (October 2010): 174–181.

Steven M. Southwick, MD, and Dennis S. Charney, MD, *Resilience: The Science of Mastering Life's Greatest Challenges* (Cambridge University Press, 2012).

Mustafa Sarkar, David Fletcher, and Daniel J. Brown, "What Doesn't Kill Me...: Adversity-Related Experiences Are Vital in the Development of Superior Olympic Performance," *Journal of Science and Medicine in Sport*, 18, no. 4 (July 2015): 475–479.

Gwen Cooper, *Homer's Odyssey* (Delacorte Press, 2009).

Paul J. Zak, "Why Inspiring Stories Make Us React: The Neuroscience of Narrative," *Cerebrum*, 2015, no. 2 (January–February 2015) (https://www.ncbi.nlm.nih.gov/pmc/articles/PMC4445577/).

Chapter 10: Supporting Mental and Emotional Well-Being

U.S. Department of Veterans Affairs, PTSD: National Center for PTSD, "How Common Is PTSD?" (https://www.ptsd.va.gov/public/ptsd-overview/basics/how-common-is-ptsd.asp).

Anxiety and Depression Association of America, "Facts & Statistics" (https://adaa.org/about-adaa/press-room/facts-statistics).

Helliwell, J., Layard, R. and Sachs, J. "World Happiness Report 2017, New York: Sustainable Development Solutions Network" (2017) (http://worldhappiness.report/ed/2017/).

Centers for Disease Control and Prevention, NCHS Data Brief No. 241 April 2016, "Increase in Suicide in the United States, 1999–2014" (https://www.cdc.gov/nchs/data/databriefs/db241.pdf).

JoAnn A. Abe, "A Longitudinal Follow-up Study of Happiness and Meaning-making," *The Journal of Positive Psychology*, 11, no. 5 (2016): 489–498. (https://www.tandfonline.com/doi/abs/10.1080/17439760.2015.1117129).

Roy F. Baumeister, Kathleen D. Vohs, Jennifer L. Aaker, and Emily N. Garbinsky, "Some Key Differences between a Happy Life and a Meaningful Life," *The Journal of Positive Psychology*, 8, no. 6 (2013) 505–516. (https://www.tandfonline.com/doi/full/10.1080/17439760.2013.830764?src=recsys).

Alfonso Sollami, Elisa Gianferrari, Manuela Alfieri, and Chiara Taffurelli, "Pet Therapy: An Effective Strategy to Care for the Elderly? An Experimental Study in a Nursing Home," *Acta Bio-medica: Atenei Parmensis*, 88, no. 1 (March 2017): 25–31.

Marguerite E. O'Haire, Noemie A. Guerin, and Alison C. Kirkham, "Animal-Assisted Intervention for Trauma: A Systematic Literature Review," *Frontiers in Psychology,* 6 (August 7, 2015) (https://www.ncbi.nlm.nih.gov/pmc/articles/PMC4528099/).

University of Buffalo News Center, "Pet-Owning Couples Are Closer, Interact More than Pet-Less Couples, UB Study Shows" (http://www.buffalo.edu/news/releases/1998/03/3479.html).

Leslie Irvine, "Animals as Lifechangers and Lifesavers," *Journal of Contemporary Ethnography,* 42, no. 1 (August 2012): 3–30.

Emma Ward-Griffin, Patrick Klaiber, Hanne K. Collins, Rhea L. Owens, Stanley Coren, and Frances S. Chen, "Petting Away Pre-exam Stress: The Effect of Therapy Dog Sessions on Student Well-being," *Stress and Health,* 34, no. 3 (August 2018): 468–473.

Attila Andics, Marta Gacsi, Tamas Farago, Anna Kis, and Adam Miklosi, "Voice-Sensitive Regions in the Dog and Human Brain Are Revealed by Comparative fMRI," *Current Biology,* 24, no. 5 (March 2014): 574–578.

Helen Brooks, Kelly Rushton, Sandra Walker, Karina Lovell, and Anne Rogers, "Ontological Security and Connectivity Provided by Pets: A Study in the Self-management of the Everyday Lives of People Diagnosed with Long-term Mental Health Condition," *BMC Psychiatry,* 16, no. 1 (December 2016): 409 (https://bmcpsychiatry.biomedcentral.com/articles/10.1186/s12888-016-1111-3).

"The Mindful Survey: The Mindful Pet?" *Mindful,* October 31, 2017 (https://www.mindful.org/mindful-survey-mindful-pet/).

Eckhart Tolle, *The Power of Now* (New World Library, 1999).

Tom Ireland, "What Does Mindfulness Meditation Do to Your Brain?" *Scientific American,* June 12, 2014 (https://blogs.scientificamerican.com/guest-blog/what-does-mindfulness-meditation-do-to-your-brain/).

Chapter 11: Fostering Children's Development

Marguerite E. O'Haire, Samantha J. McKenzie, Alan M. Beck, and Virginia Slaughter, "Social Behaviors Increase in Children with Autism in the Presence of Animals Compared to Toys," *PLOS One,* 8, no. 2 (January 2013) (http://journals.plos.org/plosone/article?id=10.1371/journal.pone.0057010).

Marguerite E. O'Haire, Samantha J. McKenzie, Alan M. Beck, and Virginia Slaughter, "Animals May Act as Social Buffers: Skin Conductance Arousal in Children with Autism Spectrum Disorder in a Social Context," *Developmental Psychobiology,* 57, no. 5 (March 2015): 584–595. (https://vet.purdue.edu/chab/ohaire/files/documents/DevPsych_2015_OHaire.pdf).

Sophie Hall, Hannah F. Wright, Annette Hames, PAWS Team, and Daniel Mills, "The Long-term Benefits of Dog Ownership in Families with Children with Autism," *Journal of Veterinary Behavior: Clinical Applications and Research,* (May–June 2016): 46–54.

American Academy of Child & Adolescent Psychiatry, "Pets and Children," May 2013 (https://www.aacap.org/AACAP/Families_and_Youth/Facts_for_Families/FFF-Guide/Pets-And-Children-075.aspx).

Pew Research, *Parenting in America,* Section 3: Parenting Approaches and Concerns, 2015 (http://www.pewsocialtrends.org/2015/12/17/3-parenting-approaches-and-concerns/).

Federal Interagency Forum on Child and Family Statistics, "America's Children: Key National Indicators of Well-Being," 2017 (https://files.eric.ed.gov/fulltext/ED577338.pdf).

National Institute of Mental Health, Statistics, "Prevalence of Any Anxiety Disorder among Adolescents" (https://www.nimh.nih.gov/health/statistics/any-anxiety-disorder.shtml#part_155096).

Ramin Mojtabai, Mark Olfson, and Beth Han, "National Trends in the Prevalence and Treatment of Depression in Adolescents and Young Adults," *Pediatrics,* 138, no. 6 (November 2016) (http://pediatrics.aappublications.org/content/early/2016/11/10/peds.2016-1878).

Centers for Disease Control and Prevention, "Autism Spectrum Disorder, Data & Statistics" (https://www.cdc.gov/ncbddd/autism/data.html).

CHADD, National Resource on ADHD, "Data and Statistics" (http://www.chadd.org/understanding-adhd/about-adhd/data-and-statistics/general-prevalence.aspx).

Kristine M. Hansen, Cathy J. Messinger, Mara M. Baun, and Mary Megel, "Companion Animals Alleviating Distress in Children," *Anthrozoos,* 12, no. 3 (1999): 142–148.

Megan Kiely Mueller and Kristina Schmid Callina, "Human-Animal Interaction as a Context for Thriving and Coping in Military-Connected Youth: The Role of Pets during Deployment," *Applied Developmental Science,* 18, no. 4 (2014): 214–223.

D. R. Ownby, C. C. Johnson, and E. L. Peterson, "Exposure to Dogs and Cats in the First Year of Life and Risk of Allergic Sensitization at 6 to 7 Years of Age," *Journal of the American Medical Association,* 288, no. 8 (August 2002): 963–972.

National Institutes of Health, "Infant Exposure to Pet and Pest Allergens May Reduce Asthma Risk," September 26, 2017 (https://www.nih.gov/news-events/nih-research-matters/infant-exposure-pet-pest-allergens-may-reduce-asthma-risk).

Megan K. Mueller "Is Human-Animal Interaction (HAI) Linked to Positive Youth Development? Initial Answer," *Applied Developmental Science,* 18, no. 1 (2014): 5–16.

Froma Walsh, "Human-Animal Bonds II: The Role of Pets in Family Systems and Family Therapy," *Family Process,* 48, no. 4 (December 2009): 481–499 (https://pdfs.semanticscholar.org/1ba0/35d468596416fec378a0c2f3091aa30477b5.pdf).

Carri Westgarth, Lynne M. Boddy, Gareth Stratton, Alexander J. German, Rosalind M. Gaskell, Karen P. Coyne, Peter Bundred, Sandra McCune, and Susan

Dawson, "Pet ownership, dog types and attachment to pets in 9–10 year old children in Liverpool, UK," *BMC Veterinary Research*, 13, no. 9 (May 2013) (https://www.ncbi.nlm.nih.gov/pmc/articles/PMC3655841/).

UC Davis, "Reading to Rover: Does It Really Help Children? Veterinary School Says, 'Yes,'" April 16, 2010 (https://www.ucdavis.edu/news/reading -rover-does-it-really-help-children-veterinary-school-says-%E2%80%98yes %E2%80%99/).

Sophie Susannah Hall, Nancy R. Gee, and Daniel Simon Mills, "Children Reading to Dogs: A Systematic Review of the Literature," *PLOS One*, 11, no. 2 (February 2016) (https://www.ncbi.nlm.nih.gov/pmc/articles/PMC4763282/).

Rebecca Purewal, Robert Christley, Katarzyna Kordas, Carol Joinson, Kerstin Meints, Nance Gee, and Carrie Westgarth, "Companion Animals and Child/ Adolescent Development: A Systematic Review of the Evidence," *International Journal of Environmental Research and Public Health*, 14, no. 3 (February 2017) (http://www.mdpi.com/1660-4601/14/3/234/htm).

Daphne Ling, Melissa Kelly, and Adele Diamond, "Human-Animal Interaction and the Development of Executive Functions," in *The Social Neuroscience of Human-Animal Interaction*, ed. Lisa S. Freund, Sandra McCune, Layla Esposito, Nancy R. Gee, and Peggy McCardle (American Psychological Association, 2016), 59.

SECTION IV: CONNECTION

Chapter 12: Enriching Relationships

Nicolas Gueguen and Serge Ciccotti, "Domestic Dogs as Facilitators in Social Inter- action: An Evaluation of Helping and Courtship Behaviors," *Anthrozoos*, 21, no. 4 (2008): 339–349 (https://www.tandfonline.com/doi/pdf/10.2752/17530370 8X371564).

Peter B. Gray, Shelly L. Volsche, Justin R. Garcia, and Helen E. Fisher, "The Roles of Pet Dogs and Cats in Human Courtship and Dating," *Anthrozoos*, 28, no. 4 (2015): 673–683 (https://www.tandfonline.com/doi/pdf/10.1080/08927936.2015 .1064216).

Anika Cloutier and Johanna Peetz, "Relationships' Best Friend: Links between Pet Ownership, Empathy, and Romantic Relationship Outcomes," *Anthrozoos*, 29, no. 3 (2016): 395–408.

Suzanne Phillips, PsyD, "Can Pets Improve Your Relationship?" PsychCentral, 2010 (https://blogs.psychcentral.com/healing-together/2010/04/can-pets-improve -your-relationship/).

Shanuti Feldman, *The Surprising Secrets of High Happy Marriages: The Little Things That Make a Big Difference* (Multnomah, 2013).

Pets of the Homeless, FAQs (https://www.petsofthehomeless.org/about-us/faqs/).

Leslie Irvine, *My Dog Always Eats First: Homeless People and Their Animals* (Lynne Rienner Publishers, Inc., 2012).

Dr. John Townsend, *Loving People: How to Love & Be Loved* (Thomas Nelson, Inc., 2008).

Chapter 13: Beyond Cats and Dogs

Julie L. Earles, Laura L. Vernon, and Jeanne P. Yetz, "Equine-Assisted Therapy for Anxiety and Posttraumatic Stress Symptoms," *Journal of Traumatic Stress*, 28 (April 2015) 149–152 (http://home.fau.edu/jearles/web/Earles,%20Vernon,%20 &%20Yetz%20(2015)%20Equine-assisted%20therapy.%20Journal%20of%20 Traumatic%20Stress.pdf).

Jessica Rossiter and Elise Matthews, "Equine-Assisted Psychotherapy (EAP) as a Valid Means of Treatment for Some Survivors of Sexual Abuse," (2011) (https:// prescottjournal.files.wordpress.com/2011/05/eapresearch1.pdf).

Janet Froeschle, "Empowering Abused Women through Equine Assisted Career Therapy," *Journal of Creativity in Mental Health*, 4, no. 2 (June 2009): 180–190.

K. Wilson, M. Buultjens, M. Monfries, and L. Karimi, "Equine-Assisted Psychotherapy for Adolescents Experiencing Depression and/or Anxiety: A Therapist's Perspective," *Clinical Child Psychology and Psychiatry*, 22, no. 1 (January 2017): 16–33.

M. Borgi, D. Loliva, S. Cerino, et al., "Effectiveness of a Standardized Equine-Assisted Therapy Program for Children with Autism Spectrum Disorder," *Journal of Autism and Developmental Disorders*, 46, no. 1 (January 2016): 1–9.

U.S. Department of Veterans Affairs, "Reining in PTSD with Equestrian Therapy," September 18, 2014 (https://www.va.gov/health/newsfeatures/2014/September/ Reining-In-PTSD-With-Equestrian-Therapy.asp).

Tufts University, "Horse Evolution over 55 Million Years," Excerpted from the Florida Museum of Natural History Fossil Horse Cybermuseum (http://chem.tufts .edu/science/evolution/horseevolution.htm).

Evening Standard, "NHS Recruits Snakes to Treat Depression," June 12, 2009 (https://www.standard.co.uk/news/nhs-recruits-snakes-to-treat-depression -6764438.html).

Diane C. Lade and *South Florida Sun Sentinel*, "Therapy Turtle Helps Kids Come out of Their Shell," *Washington Post*, March 18, 2012.

Gail F. Melson, *Where the Wild Things Are* (Harvard University Press, 2001), 83.

B. J. Park, Y. Tsuetsugu, T. Kasetani, T. Kagawa, and Y. Miyazaki, "The Physiological Effects of Shinrin-yoku (taking in the forest atmosphere or forest bathing): Evidence from Field Experiments in 24 Forests across Japan," *Environmental Health and Preventive Medicine*, 15, no. 1 (January 2010): 18–26.

John M. Zelenski, Raelyne L. Dopko, and Colin A. Capaldi, "Cooperation Is in Our Nature: Nature Exposure May Promote Cooperative and Environmentally

Sustainable Behavior," *Journal of Environment Psychology*, 42 (June 2015): 24–31 (https://www.sciencedirect.com/science/article/pii/S0272494415000195).

Simon Maken, "Feeling Awe May Be Good for Our Health," *Scientific American*, September 1, 2015. (https://www.scientificamerican.com/article/feeling-awe-may-be-good-for-our-health/)

Paul K. Piff, Pia Dietze, Matthew Feinberg, Daniel M. Stancato, and Dacher Keltner, "Awe, the Small Self, and Prosocial Behavior," *Journal of Personality and Social Psychology*, 108, no. 6 (June 2015): 883–899 (https://gratefulness.org/content/uploads/2016/02/Awe-the-Small-Self-and-Prosocial-Behavior.pdf).

SpaceQuotations.com, Looking Back at Earth Quotes (http://www.spacequotations.com/earth.html).

Chapter 14: Discovering Purpose

American Express, NEWS, "New Study: Americans Say Road to Success Now Paved More with Fulfillment Than Wealth," May 15, 2013 (http://about.americanexpress.com/news/pr/2013/americans-say-road-to-success-fulfillment.aspx).

Viktor Frankl, *Man's Search for Meaning*, (Beacon Press, 2006). Originally published in 1946.

The Dalai Lama and Arthur C. Brooks, "Dalai Lama: Behind Our Anxiety, the Fear of Being Unneeded," *New York Times*, November 4, 2016 (https://www.nytimes.com/2016/11/04/opinion/dalai-lama-behind-our-anxiety-the-fear-of-being-unneeded.html).

Emily Esfahani, *The Power of Meaning: Crafting a Life That Matters* (Crown, 2017).

Andrew Bloomfield, *Call of the Cats: What I Learned about Life and Love from a Feral Colony* (New World Library, 2016).

Larry Dossey, MD, *One Mind: How Our Individual Mind Is Part of a Greater Consciousness and Why It Matters* (Hay House, 2013).

Barbara Fredrickson, PhD, *Love 2.0: Finding Happiness and Health in Moments of Connection* (Plume, Reprint edition, 2013), 16.

Lydia Warren, "'She's the one who taught me what love is': Singer Fiona Apple's Moving Eulogy to Dying Dog as She Postpones Tour to Be with Her," *Daily Mail*, November 21, 2012 (http://www.dailymail.co.uk/news/article-2236289/Fiona-Apples-extraordinary-eulogy-dying-dog-cancels-tour-her.html). Used with permission from Fiona Apple.

About the Author and Collaborator

Carol Novello is founder of Mutual Rescue™, a national initiative focused on changing the conversation from "people *or* animals" to "people *and* animals" with the aim of elevating the cause of animal welfare. Through authentic storytelling, Mutual Rescue presents compelling evidence that when people adopt homeless animals, their own lives are often dramatically transformed in positive ways as well. *Eric & Peety*, the first Mutual Rescue film, has been viewed more than 100 million times across the globe. Mutual Rescue also drives engagement at the local level by encouraging people to take shelter dogs on outings in the community through Doggy Day Out programs. Carol is now expanding the initiative into a national nonprofit brand to bring new funding into the sector through corporate sponsorships in order to advance both the practice of shelter medicine and collaboration between animal welfare and human services organizations across the United States.

For nearly a decade, Carol served as president of Humane Society Silicon Valley (HSSV), one of the largest privately funded animal rescue organizations in the San Francisco Bay Area. Through her leadership, HSSV became a "model shelter"—the first organization ever to meet all guidelines set forth by the Association of Shelter Veterinarians. Her work at HSSV resulted in significant increases in the rescue organization's adoption numbers, save rate, and the number of animals receiving extended care.

Previously, Carol was a senior executive at Intuit, Inc., where she held numerous positions including president of MasterBuilder

Software, vice president/general manager of QuickBooks Online, vice president—marketing for QuickBooks and Small Business Products and Services, and vice president/general manager of Quicken and QuickBooks Checks, Forms, and Supplies.

Carol has an MBA from Harvard Business School and a BA in economics and English from Dickinson College. She has been recognized with the prestigious Maddie Hero Award for innovation and leadership in the animal welfare sector, as an honoree at the Fifty Years of Women at Harvard Business School celebration in Northern California, named a Woman of Influence by *San Jose Business Journal,* and inducted into Marquis Who's Who in America. Her family includes two rescue tuxedo cats: Bode and Herbie. She lives in Serenbe, a community outside of Atlanta, Georgia.

Ginny Graves specializes in bringing wellness, mental health, fitness, and medical reporting to life for general audiences. An award-winning journalist, she has spent her thirty-year career crafting narratives about people and the issues that fascinate, worry, beset, and inspire them. She is best known for her massive trove of in-depth magazine features, which have enlivened the pages and been touted on the covers of O *The Oprah Magazine, Vogue, Elle, Glamour, Runner's World, TIME, Cosmopolitan, Reader's Digest,* and *National Geographic Adventure.* She has also collaborated on a number of books, including *Bringing Home the Bacon: Making Marriage Work When She Makes More Money.* When she's not meeting deadlines, she's usually on the trails or at the beach with her three dogs near her home in Fairfax, California.